Everything About Alzheimer's Disease

101 Questions and Answers

Adrian Stănescu, MD

To my mother, who discretely guided our steps towards medicine - with love and passion that you have laid upon us in a lifetime, a dream which has come true through your beloved children.

Many thanks, also, to my wife and my children who constantly supported me in all my efforts in the realm of medicine.

I would like to acknowledge the support of my mentors in the medical activity - in chronological order - Dr. Ioana Mihalache, Dr. Anca Domocoș, Professor Luiza Spiru, MD, Professor Alexandru Șerbănescu, MD.

The Author

September 2017

Contents

1. How does normal aging of the brain manifest itself? — 15
2. What is dementia? — 16
3. What are the causes of dementia? — 18
4. What is Alzheimer's disease? — 19
5. Who discovered Alzheimer's disease? — 21
6. When is the Alzheimer's diagnosis certain? — 22
7. Are Alzheimer dementia and Alzheimer's disease the same thing? — 23
8. What are the stages of Alzheimer's disease? — 24
9. How can the preclinical stage of Alzheimer's disease be diagnosed? — 26
10. What is vascular dementia? — 28
11. What is mixed dementia? — 30
12. What are the other types of dementia? — 31
13. Could we know from the beginning what type of dementia the patient has? — 35
14. Which is the more dangerous type of dementia: Alzheimer's or vascular? — 38
15. How long does Alzheimer's disease last? What about Alzheimer dementia? — 39
16. How long does vascular dementia last? What about other types of dementia? — 40
17. Can Alzheimer's disease occur at an age as early as 40? What about Alzheimer dementia? — 41
18. Will I suffer from Alzheimer's disease if my mother does? — 42
19. Are there any tests to detect the risk of getting Alzheimer's disease? — 43
20. How common is Alzheimer's disease? How about dementia in general? — 46
21. Is the frequency of this disease higher in more developed countries? — 47

22.	Are there any differences between different races in the frequency of Alzheimer's disease?	48
23.	Can Alzheimer's disease be prevented? What about Alzheimer dementia?	49
24.	What are the structural changes in the brain in dementia?	50
25.	What are the risk factors for dementias?	53
26.	Is diabetes a risk factor in Alzheimer dementia?	54
27.	Is hypertension a risk factor in dementia?	56
28.	Is smoking a risk factor in dementia?	57
29.	Is there any relationship between stress and dementia?	58
30.	Are people with more education more prone to Alzheimer dementia?	59
31.	Can high cholesterol in the blood cause Alzheimer's disease?	60
32.	Can thyroid disease cause a form of dementia?	60
33.	Can heart disease cause dementia?	62
34.	What is mild cognitive impairment? What about subjective cognitive impairment?	64
35.	How can we find out whether the mild cognitive impairment precedes dementia?	69
36.	What are the biomarkers of Alzheimer's disease? Where and when do they occur?	70
37.	Why is the early diagnosis of Alzheimer's disease important?	78
38.	Can we improve our memory?	80
39.	What is cognitive reserve?	82
40.	Is there a cognitive frailty syndrome of the elderly?	84
41.	What is cognitive stimulation?	86
42.	What are the simplest cognitive stimulation exercises?	89
43.	Until what stage of the illness can the cognitive stimulation be used?	92
44.	Do physical exercises help improve	93

	memory?	
45.	What are the limits of physical exercise in dementia?	98
46.	What are the costs of care in Alzheimer dementia?	100
47.	What are the stages of Alzheimer's disease? What about Alzheimer dementia?	101
48.	Can we quickly assess the stage of the disease?	102
49.	What is the first typical sign of Alzheimer's?	104
50.	If you start forgetting in your fifties, does it mean that one will develop Alzheimer's?	106
51.	What are the clinical manifestations of the mild form of Alzheimer dementia?	107
52	What are the clinical manifestations of the medium form of Alzheimer dementia?	109
53.	What are the clinical manifestations of the severe form of Alzheimer dementia?	110
54.	Can clinical manifestations vary depending on the time of day?	111
55.	Does sexual desire diminish or disappear in patients with dementia?	113
56.	Currently, are there reversible or curable types of dementia?	115
57.	How early should the treatment of this illness begin?	123
58.	Who are the doctors who can help?	126
59.	What tests must be done first? What about later?	128
60.	Are the imagistic tests mandatory from the beginning?	135
61.	Should environmental changes for patients with dementia be avoided?	137
62.	Can a patient have dementia and depression at the same time?	138
63.	May depression precede dementia?	139
64.	What are the most common behavioral disorders in dementia?	140
65.	When can behavioral disorders occur in the	

	illness?	144
66.	Can the caregivers' behavior influence the illness?	145
67.	How can we help caregivers cope with the situation?	146
68.	Can impaired sleep influence the illness?	147
69.	What are the problems which the patient with dementia can cause?	149
70.	Can we delay its progression?	150
71.	When should we consult a doctor for the first time?	151
72.	What should the doctor look for on the first appointment?	152
73.	At what interval should the patient be re-evaluated?	155
74.	Are there any signs which can confirm the diagnosis of Alzheimer dementia?	156
75.	Should the patient with dementia be treated from the beginning?	157
76.	Are there any drugs that cure this illness?	157
77.	Should certain medications be avoided in the treatment of dementia?	158
78.	Are there other remedies in Alzheimer dementia?	159
79.	What are the classes of medications used to treat dementia?	161
80.	How frequent are the side effects of the administered medicine?	168
81.	Are there currently any new medications in research phase?	171
82.	What are the complications of an antipsychotic treatment and what should we do?	173
83.	How should we act if the patient is agitated or even violent?	175
84.	What type of care should be given in the terminal phase?	177
85.	Should drug therapy be discontinued in the terminal phase?	182

86.	Is institutionalization compulsory in the terminal phase?	*183*
87.	How should we behave around a terminal patient?	*183*
88.	Do all patients reach the stage of bed confinement?	*184*
89.	What are the complications of bed confinement?	*185*
90.	Is there a diet which protects against Alzheimer's disease?	*186*
91.	How do we assess the nutritional status of patients with dementia?	*189*
92.	What are the investigations in the nutritional status evaluation of Alzheimer's?	*192*
93.	What is the proper nutrition in Alzheimer dementia?	*193*
94.	How is proper hydration achieved for a patient with dementia?	*200*
95.	Can dementia be cured with a natural treatment?	*203*
96.	Is the early diagnosis of Alzheimer's disease useful and ethical?	*204*
97.	Should we be afraid of dementia?	*205*
98.	Can we accept the harsh reality of a dementia diagnosis?	*207*
99.	Can we live through this illness with dignity?	*208*
100.	What are the myths and misconceptions about Alzheimer's disease?	*209*
101.	Are there miracles in Alzheimer's disease?	*213*

Foreword

Imagine a world in which there are no illnessses like cancer or Alzheimer's....

Surely, it would be much less sadness and truly huge sums of money spent on the care of patients with these illnesses in terminal stages might be used for other useful purposes like health, education and human civilization in general.

Do you think this is impossible? If we refer to short periods of time, you might be right. But what would have thought the 18th century people about the possibility of remote communication through a device (first the telegraph, afterwards the telephone). Or, the 19th century people about the ability to be transported in "flying machines" at extraordinary speeds of hundreds of kilometers per hour at altitudes of over 10,000 meters above the Earth. Or would the early 20th century "little people" who were barely familiar with inventions such as the light bulb or car thought – if they would have lived long enough – they would be contemporaries with the first man to set foot on the moon?

Do you see what I mean? Nothing, absolutely nothing is impossible! We already live in a world of holograms, drones, nanorobots and other inventions which did not exist twenty years before. Children elaborate nuclear reactors in school labs... A man "jumped" in the stratosphere (from an altitude of 30 km) and landed on Earth safely. We talk about artificial intelligence – biocomputers – or teleportation as about some natural things which in a moment might become part of our life.

This is the reason medicine will also make incredible "jumps" in future decades, similar to the stratosphere jump of Felix Baumgartner, and illnesses like cancer or Alzheimer dementia will be part of the history of medicine. But until then, what do we do? Because there will be millions of people who will suffer from these illnesses until the discovery of complete curative treatments. But until then, will we be waiting in a resigned attitude? What is the solution? I'll give an answer as simple as it is natural... KNOWLEDGE. But this must happen within the "masses" of the population. And for this reason, the tools to be used should be standard and easy to understand. I will not use sophisticated terms which can confuse the reader, but by using layman's terms.

This book is a more elaborate continuation of the first guide published five years ago, in a small edition *What should you know about Alzheimer's?*

This book is trying to gain the attention of those who are facing this endemic that has encompassed all mankind and that the World Health Organization has called "the medical terror of the 21st century", and also of those who want to be informed or to learn about what can be done at this time to keep away from this unseen enemy.

The structure of this book is in the form of 101 questions, which I have most commonly encountered in my medical practice in this area (over 15 years and a total of several thousand patients), questions asked either by caregivers – as I will refer here to those who deal directly with patients – or even the patients themselves who are eager to find solutions to their problems. The language I use is easy to understand by the reader, without affecting the scientific content of the information, but concentrating this information to its essence. Sometimes, the term "Alzheimer's" will be directly used, as more recently practiced in scientific presentations in order to simplify the transmitted message.

Immediately after this "Foreword" all these questions will be lined up so that you, the reader, can go directly to the question whose answer you are looking for! This way, the book can be read easily and you can skip to the items of interest, depending on your desire to acquire more or less information about "Alzheimer" as the entire cognitive pathology is now known.

The fluent reading of this book will also present some repetitions of ideas in the context of the presented questions, basically giving answer to the same topic, which will ultimately help in understanding some concepts considered important by the author.

I wish you an easy and very useful reading experience!

1. How does normal aging of the brain manifest itself?

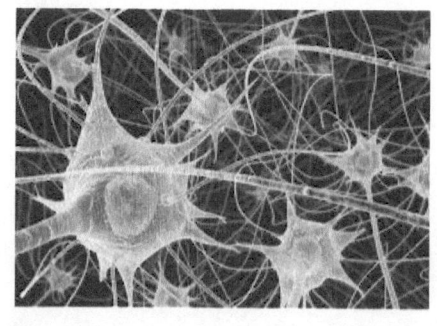
Senescence (aging) is not an illness; it is a physiological process, even if it is usually unecessarily associated with different illnesses. Various physiological changes appear to be directly related to aging, but many older people preserve their functional capacity even with all this organic degeneration. Today, the age of 60-65 years is considered as the threshold for old age. As life

expectancy increases, this threshold will also be changed soon.

The brain, like any other organ, undergoes aging, seemingly normal, progressively and constantly. It can be equated with the physiological loss of neurons and synapses (links) among neurons that start at a young age but also, with some changes of neurohormones secreted in the brain. All these lead to changes in voluntary normal human processes as coordinated by the brain (cognitive, motor activity, releasing hormones).

As a result of the brain's normal aging, changes may appear in the reaction time of remembering certain events or in more complex processes such as abstract thinking or decision making, but not severe enough to cause impairment of the individual's daily activities.

This can be confused with dementia syndromes that have a similar onset; the difference between the two entities could only be recognized by the specialists, following specific, standardized assessments and repeated evaluation.

2. What is dementia?

Dementia is a syndrome characterized by deterioration of intellectual functions (cognitive and emotional skills) severe enough to interfere with daily activities and quality of life occurring in a conscious patient.

As we can see, dementia is not an illness. "Dementia" is an general term which circumscribes, first of all, disorders of brain functions such as memory problems, spatial and temporal disorientation, confusion, impairment of complex brain activities (abstract thinking, decision making), but especially affecting the daily activity of an ordinary person.

We say that dementia is a syndrome because it meets the definition of being a group of signs and symptoms that occur in particular pathologies.

If we follow the specialty literature, signs and specific symptoms of dementia are intertwined, unlike other syndromes in which they are clearly differentiated. Thus, among the signs and symptoms of dementia, we find forgetting recently learned information, changes in planning and solving problems such as handling money, using one's phone and remembering phone numbers previously known by the patient, etc.

Dementia is incorrectly defined as a process of aging – "senilization" – which is rather common for normal brain aging but that does not affect a person's daily activity.

The signs and symptoms may vary greatly, but at least two of these must be significantly affected to meet the criteria for dementia:

• Memory

• Language and communication

• Visual perception

• Attention

• Reasoning

Usually, dementia is progressive and its early diagnosis increases the chances to slow down its evolution by initiating specific treatments which allow the early planning of life.

3. What are the causes of dementia?

The causes of signs and symptoms in dementia are the impairments of various neural structures which interfere with their ability to interrelate (communication between them). These structures with different localization (Appendix 1) are designed to control different intellectual functions such as learning (ability to add new information to that already known), saving (data storage) and reasoning (sorting and using the information). Besides, other brain structures are also affected as, for instance, those coordinating movements.

The causes of dementia causes remain unknown despite the advances made in the last 10-15 years of research. Structural changes occurring in neurons, manifested by abnormal deposits of peptides (accumulation of an extracellular substance called β - amyloid or an intracellular protein ζ (tau) in the form of neurofibrillary tangles) seem to be secondary to the primary causes of developing dementia. Moreover, given the variety of manifestations of dementias and the multitude of dementia syndromes, it is more likely that there is a complexity of causes.

Some authors assimilate these causes with risk factors (such as vascular risk factors) but perhaps this can only accelerate the illness.

4. What is Alzheimer's disease?

Alzheimer's disease is a progressive neurodegenerative disorder characterized by destruction of nerve cells, consisting in a long asymptomatic phase – the patient does not show any sign related to memory and reasoning (10-15 years), followed by clinical stage (other 8-10 years) with specific events around cognitive, behavioral disorders, (memory loss, impaired reasoning, etc). These points in time are the result of statistical studies and do not necessarily represent the evolution of every patient – **"There are patients, not illnesses."**

Thus, one can see that a person suffering from this illness and passes away because of it at 75, has probably had its stigmas starting at 50-55. When referring to people with he severe form of the illness at 60 years (cases quite rare, but numerically increasing lately), we realize that in certain circumstances (to which we will refer extensively in this book), the diagnosis could be made right around the age of

35-40 years. That's why persons at risk, having parents or grandparents with Alzheimer dementia, would require early screening in the "young adult" periods.

Regarding the clinical stage, this is divided into mild cognitive impairment (MCI) and Alzheimer dementia (AD) itself. The difference between the two stages is that in the case of cognitive deficit (which is now regarded as part of mild neurocognitive disorder according to the latest specialty classification – DSM V, Appendix 2), there is a lack of impairment in daily activities, as it is the case in dementia.

Alzheimer's disease is the most common form of dementia for people over 65 years.

5. Who discovered Alzheimer's disease?

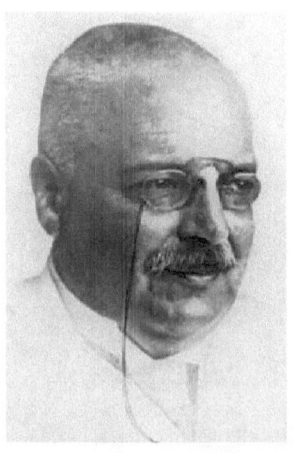

Alzheimer's disease was discovered over 100 years ago (in 1906) by the German physician Alois Alzheimer who presented the case of a woman aged only 51, who suffered both from memory and behavioral disorders. Necrological histologic examination of the neurons revealed the presence of amyloid plaques and neurofibrillary tangles characteristic of this illness.

The recognition of Alois Alzheimer's merit is due to Emil Kraepelin who mentioned the illness, under this name, in his treatise on psychiatry in 1910.

As later it has been considered that the first patient diagnosis was actually different, Alzheimer's role was at least to signal a new category of neurodegenerative illnesses that are manifested especially by memory loss.

6. *When is the Alzheimer's diagnosis certain?*

Until recently it has been said that a certain diagnosis of Alzheimer's disease can only be made at the stage of autopsy by examining the patient's neurons. Following the occurrence of combined tests that increase the diagnostic possibility above 95%, one can say that the perspective on this subject has changed.

A comprehensive evaluation to establish a probable diagnosis of Alzheimer's disease includes:

• Medical history obtained from the patient or caregiver.

• Medical tests to rule out other causes.

• Imaging tests (preferably MRI brain, but the brain scan is also useful. Now, whenever possible, the PET is recommended (see Question 60).

• Specific humoral tests (blood and cerebrospinal fluid) (see question 19).

• Psychometric testing through cognitive tests which evaluate cognitive function including short-term memory, attention, spatial and temporal orientation, language, abstract thinking, executive functions and the ability to make decisions (see Question 59).

7. Are Alzheimer dementia and Alzheimer's disease the same thing?

Within the population, but sometimes even in the medical world, there is a confusion between Alzheimer's disease and dementia. As we emphasized in the previous questions,

Alzheimer's disease includes the Alzheimer dementia stage when symptoms and specific signs are severe enough to interfere with daily activities and the patient depends on another person to live a life as close as possible to normal.

Unfortunately, Alzheimer's disease is revealed only in the stage of dementia (and even worse, in its medium and severe forms), when pathological changes in neurons are irreversible and treatments are (at least so far) only symptomatic (to improve the clinical status of the patient).

On the other hand, due to external factors or other simultaneous morbidities, it is possible for this stigma of Alzheimer's disease to be observed at necropsy, before the patient having developed dementia itself. If these histopathological examinations were done systematically, one might be able to find a much larger number of potential patients with Alzheimer's disease who remained undiagnosed in their lifetime.

In degenerative demantias, according to certain older statistics, Alzheimer's dementia is the most frequent, being responsible for 60-80% of them. Recent research, based on histopathological studies of the post-mortem brain, increased the percentage of mixed demantias (especialy the mixed type between Alzheimer's and vascular), consequently decreasing the percentage of Alzheimer's dementias in this classification of the dementias' etiology.

8. What are the stages of Alzheimer's disease?

According to a 2011 classification, Alzheimer's disease has three distinct stages:

• **The preclinical stage**, where there are no specific symptoms of dementia, but certain biomarkers in the cerebrospinal fluid can be identified.

• **The mild cognitive deficit stage**, which includes specific symptoms which are not severe enough to affect daily activities.

• **The active illness stage**, known as Alzheimer dementia, when the patient requires support for daily activities and subsequently permanent surveillance.

From 2015, the DSM V classification has entered into force, Alzheimer dementia being divided into two major classes:

- **Minor neurocognitive disorder** which includes mild cognitive impairment and a light form of dementia.

- **Major neurocognitive disorder** which includes medium and severe forms of dementia.

The main goal of this new classification is to eliminate the "dementia" stigma from classifications, to a better and more compliant approach of the patient and his family to the prescribed treatment. On the other hand, a patient with mild cognitive impairment, which will not necessarily lead to dementia, will be assigned to class "minor neurocognitive disorder" and will allow – on a case-by-case basis -, even the administration of specific treatment in the presence of risk factors which are likely involved in the development of dementia (a patient whose cognitive deficit is associated with hypertension, diabetes and hypercholesterolemia).

The new DSM V classification of memory problems also takes into account cognitive domains wich are rather intuited than named in the previous classification, such as complex attention, executive functions and social cognition – see Appendix 2, drawing attention to rather hardly perceptible changes which are harder to perceive by laymen.

9. How can the preclinical stage of Alzheimer's disease be diagnosed?

The preclinical phase (or stage) is considered favorable to the prevention of dementia itself.

In a study made by an American working group, this phase is divided into three stages:

Stage 1 – characterized by the presence of asymptomatic amyloid (see Question 36).

Stage 2 – adds the presence of the synaptic dysfunction and neurodegeneration.

Stage 3 – adds the presence of some subtle and inconstant cognitive changes to the changes from stage 2.

This classification is very helpful, yet heterogeneous, by using both clinical and structural data.

In this study framework, coordinated by dr. Knopman from the Mayo University and Guy Mc Khann from John Hopkins University School of Medicine in the United States in 2012 on 2,000 subjects, two stages were added: stage O with "cognitively normal" subjects without specific biomarkers and the "The stand-alone category" stage (TSAC), with subjects who present normal biomarkers for amyloid but other types of dementia than Alzheimer dementia. The results were as follows:

- 43 % stage 0

- 16 % stage 1

- 12% stage 2

- 3% stage 3

- 23 % stage TSAC

The results were surprising and they show a possible preclinical stage in about 30% of the population, that is, potential patients who will develop Alzheimer dementia during their lifetime. If this study is correlated with the fact that in the population over 85 years almost one third develop dementia, we can conclude that the study is consistent with reality.

10. What is vascular dementia?

> Vascular dementia is classically described as a cognitive disorder with sudden onset and gradual deterioration caused by brain damage secondary to a decreased blood flow which deprives neurons of nutrients and oxygen.

According to some authors, the neurocognitive disorders are correlated with the degree of vascular brain damage. Vascular risk factors (hypertension, high levels of blood cholesterol, smoking, diabetes or glucose intolerance) increase the risk of vascular dementia.

Clinical manifestations vary depending on the affected brain area. In the case of a "mini-stroke" – i.e. small strokes – which is expressed in brain tomography as a "cerebral lacunar state", the evolution may be slow, similar to that of Alzheimer dementia. Common symptoms in vascular dementia are:

• Confusion

• Disorders of attention and concentration

• Excitement and anxiety especially at sunset (sundowning phenomenon) and night

- Complex impairment of the thinking functions, as organization, planning and decision making

- Disorders of recent memory, usually occur later, in contrast to Alzheimer dementia occurring after the onset

- Spastic gaits

- Inadequate laughing and crying

- Incontinence

- Depression

Besides cerebral infarction, which represents the classical cause, there are other chronic illnesses of the blood vessels in the brain such as lupus erythematosus, vasculitis, cerebral hemorrhage or temporal arteritis which can cause vascular dementia.

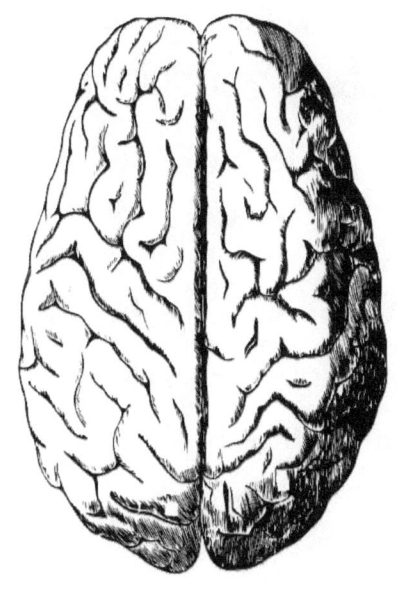

11. What is mixed dementia?

Mixed dementia is the pathological condition of the brain in which changes which are specific to different types of dementia occur simultaneously. The most common type of mixed dementia is one that combines elements of the Alzheimer's type dementia with vascular elements.

According to some authors – also confirmed by autopsy data (post-mortem histopathology) – mixed dementia would be more common than vascular dementia. It is also one of the reasons why the new DSM V classification considers the clinical criterion a main diagnostic criterion, separating major and minor neurocognitive disorders and leaving the histopathological type of dementia on the second place.

On the other hand, another study showed that 94% of people who were diagnosed with Alzheimer dementia showed specific alterations particular to vascular dementia when the autopsy examination was performed. The higher the age of onset, the more probable the mixed dementia is.

Any patient who shows signs of minor neurocognitive disorder should be subject to a complex evaluation, including humoral and imagistic evaluation, in order not to misclassify it either as degenerative or vascular dementia, without first verifying if it is a mixed dementia which, naturally, can be approached differently.

12. What are the other types of dementia?

In a simple topographical classification, dementias are cortical and subcortical, based on the affected area of the central nervous system.

Cortical dementias are the most common (Alzheimer's, vascular dementia or multi-infarct and the combination of these two types) and, as we previously mentioned (see Questions 2, 10 and 11), they are characterized mainly by memory, language, numerical calculation disorders associated with apraxia and agnosia signs (see Question 2).

In contrast, subcortical dementias (dementia in Parkinson's disease, Huntington's chorea and progressive supranuclear palsy, which affect predominantly the basal ganglia) are characterized by motility disorders from the onset, involuntary movements, slowness of thought processes (bradypsychia), and sometimes loss of initiative, and usually late in its evolution – depression.

In the most important treatise of neurology, *Principles of Neurology* published under the coordination of the great neuroscientist R. Adams, over 50 possible causes of dementia are listed.

In decreasing order of frequency, dementia types are:

- Alzheimer dementia (see Question 4).

- Vascular dementia (see Question 10).

- Dementia with Lewy bodies

- Frontotemporal Dementia

    - Other irreversible dementia (subcortical dementia)

- Reversible dementia (see Question 55)

As shown in Appendix 3, we can see that cognition is impaired in time in all 3 most common types of dementia, with a slow progression in Alzheimer, in stages, in vascular dementia and sometimes accompanied by improvement of cognition in dementia with Lewy bodies. The 3 types of dementia together with the mixed types resulting from their combination cover over 90% of the encoutered dementia cases.

Dementia with Lewy bodies (Lewy Body Dementia – DLB) is characterized by the presence of Lewy bodies – abnormal protein aggregation (synuclein and ubiquitin) in neurons – found in post-mortem histopathology. This type of dementia may begin clinically in three different ways:

• Cognitive impairments like those of Alzheimer dementia but fluctuating, impaiment of attention and of the "state of alertness", then visual hallucinations, behavioral disorders during sleep such as the "REM sleep behavior disorder", severe adverse reactions to antipsychotics,

• Walking disorders erroneously attributed to Parkinson's disease, which are followed later on by dementia,

• Psychiatric symptoms specific to the onset.

Sometimes sleep disorders may precede the onset of dementia by decades!

Frontotemporal dementia (FTD) is characterized by progressive loss of neurons (especially the "spindle neurons") with a frontal and/or a temporal location.

Previously, it has been said that 20% of dementia would be frontotemporal. With the progress of the imaging evaluation it has been proven that this share is specific to the so-called early dementias (occurring before 60 years), being much rarer in general casuistry (as dementia with Lewy bodies).

Symptomatology is characterized by personality disorders, lack of inhibition (including sexually), apathy or on the contrary, anxiety, stereotypes and preserving cognition in the beginning. Unlike other dementias, hallucinations are extremely rare. Recently, researchers have described frontotemporal dementia in association with Amyotrophic Lateral Sclerosis (ALS) whereby the nerves that coordinate voluntary movements are being impacted.

Subcortical dementias are rare dementias which can accompany cortical dementias or be stand-alone. Symptomatology is characterized by bradyphrenia (psychomotor slowing processes), perseverance, deficit of executive functions but the patient is oriented visually and spatially, retains most of the language and has only a mild memory impairment. Neurological signs of the primary disease are also present.

Reversible dementias are a special category of dementia, unfortunately underdiagnosed (see Question 56). Their diagnosis is very important because the respective entities can be treated, especially if the diagnosis is made on time.

13. Could we know from the beginning what type of dementia the patient has?

Once established, dementia is highlighted by separate symptoms. By definition, in order to diagnose dementia, these symptoms must be severe enough to affect the individual's daily activities. If the person solves his daily business independently, even if he has some symptoms of dementia, one can not talk about its presence (yet). One can talk about a pre-dementia or about a mild memory disorder which can either lead or not to a dementia.

Depending on the type of dementia, symptoms have a specific rate and a certain graduality in their appearance and presence. Thus, recent memory impairment in Alzheimer dementia is the first symptom (in most cases) and its deterioration is gradual and slow. In vascular dementia, other symptoms can occur initially (different movement disorders), but the deterioration of cognitive functions (not only memory but also other intellectual functions) is often in a "plateau" stage, meaning both stagnation stages and then rapid deterioration. On the other hand, in dementia with Lewy bodies, the memory and other cognitive functions have a leaping, fast evolution, without stationary phases (Appendix 3).

On the other hand, all suspected dementia syndrome should entail a standardized psychometric assessment and a set of tests in order to exclude certain rare types of dementia caused by certain pathological conditions (deficiency of vitamin B12 and/or folic acid, vitamin B1, vitamin PP or B3, hypothyroidism, HIV-AIDS, syphilis, Creutzfeld-Jakobs dementia, intoxication with certain substances - aluminum, etc.) or some pseudodementia (usually a severe depression specific to someone with chronical melancholy, primary or secondary (metastatic) brain tumors, pronounced hypoxia from severe heart disease and respiratory disease, hepatic encephalopathy, normal pressure hydrocephalus, cerebral hematoma – (usually subdural, posttraumatic) and many other causes.

Once diagnosed and treated, all these pathological conditions can cause partial or total reversibility of the dementia syndrome, being part of the so-called "reversible dementia". It is therefore very important that as soon as one suspects the presence of dementia, the differential diagnosis be made, treating immediately (if possible) the primary cause of the cognitive impairment. Thus, determination of vitamin B12, folic acid, thyroid hormones and regulators thyroid (T3, T4, TSH), serotonin levels (for depression) in blood, the presence of bacteria or some metals in high quantities (lead, iron, aluminum, copper) and performing imaging tests (brain, liver, etc.) are necessary since the suspicion of a dementia syndrome.

14. Which is the more dangerous type of dementia: Alzheimer's or vascular?

They say that "each patient experiences illness in his own way."

Unfortunately, there is no curable treatment in neurodegenerative dementias, either in Alzheimer dementia, vascular dementia or other types (fronto-temporal, and subcortical Lewy bodies).

The average length of survival in Alzheimer's disease, once the symptoms appear (that is the mild cognitive impairment stage when not all the criteria for the diagnosis of dementia are met, meaning that the patient's daily activity is not affected) is about 8 years.

This varies, from individual to individual, between 3 and 20 years. It depends on the age at onset and on the presence of associated illnesses (co-morbidities), such as severe illnesses affecting the heart, lung, kidney, cancer, etc.

In vascular dementia, which occurs secondary to a stroke or to small insidious strokes, the survival duration is shorter – 5 years.

In most cases death occurs after a new stroke or a heart attack.

As we said before, the pathological examination often reveals signs of both types of dementia so one can say that the average length of survival is 5-8 years.

> We can conclude that both types of dementia are equally serious, having a critical prognosis.

15. How long does Alzheimer's disease last? What about Alzheimer dementia?

Alzheimer's disease and Alzheimer dementia are different entities. (see Question 7)

Duration of survival in Alzheimer dementia is approximately 8 years (see Question 14) but it depends on the age at which specific symptomatology began.

According to some authors, the mild cognitive impairment stage that precedes the Alzheimer dementia, would take in average 2-3 years.

Finally, the first stage of Alzheimer's disease, completely asymptomatic, in which just the biomarkers of the disease are present, could last 15-20 years – see Question 4.

If you add up these values, we can say that the evolution of an Alzheimer's type neurodegenerative illness can reach the maximum period of 30 years.

16. How long does vascular dementia last? What about other types of dementia?

"Pure" vascular dementia lasts about five years from its onset. It accompanies a constituted focal stroke, sequel or small strokes that went unnoticed, but which can be highlighted by imaging methods (CT cerebral tomography, magnetic resonance imaging).

Dementia with Lewy bodies lasts about 5-7 years. Its evolution depends on proper treatment of hallucinations (severe side effects when taking neuroleptics) or fallings appearance (sudden drop in blood pressure, similar to the mechanism that occurs in Parkinson's disease).

Frontotemporal Dementia, from the appearance of the first symptoms, lasts between 6 and 8 years, but survival can last between 2 and 20 years.

17. Can Alzheimer's disease occur at an age as early as 40? What about Alzheimer dementia?

Certainly, the biomarkers of Alzheimer's disease (see Question 36) can be highlighted around the age of 40 for those patients who would develop an early Alzheimer dementia, if they would be checked systematically. Unfortunately, the high cost of such investigations does not allow such an approach yet.

As for Alzheimer dementia, the final stage of Alzheimer's disease, in which the symptoms are severe enough to cause damage to the patient's daily activity, it occurs at the earliest – rarely – around the age of 50. Statistically, Alzheimer dementia often occurs around the age of 70.

18. Will I suffer from Alzheimer's disease if my mother does?

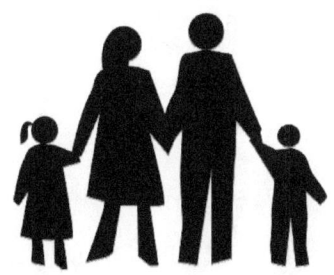

Children of patients with Alzheimer dementia (or other

types of dementia) are often worried that they will also suffer from Alzheimer's disease. The frequency of Alzheimer's disease hereditary transmission is very low, about 1-5%, according to different authors. In these rare cases, the illness usually develops much earlier. Three genes have been identified: APP, PS1 and PS2 and which are associated to the early onset of the hereditary Alzheimer dementia.

Actually, age is the most important factor in Alzheimer's disease, for the individuals who will have old age dementia there is no difference between those who had parents or grandparents with dementia and those who did not have Alzheimer's disease in the family.

Another aspect is that, in most case, either the eating habits are being inherited within the family or a deficient diet is common to several generations when children, parents and grandparents live together.

19. *Are there any tests to detect the risk of getting Alzheimer's disease?*

The human body is coordinated by the activity of its genome, which consists of about 100,000 different genes, each serving to produce and to encode proteins with different functions in the body.

Living organisms have the same biochemically genetic material: the double-stranded helix structure of DNA, which contains four bases – adenine, guanine, cytosine and thiamine (DNA found in all nucleated cells). Deleting a DNA sequence (or even a single base pair) causes genetic mutations and gives the probability of a genetic illness.

Some illnesses are caused by a single gene modification; others are determined by a combination of mutant genes.

The most common genetic illnesses caused by a single gene modification are: hyperlipidemia, hypercholesterolemia, otosclerosis, polycystic kidney illness, Huntington's illness, neurofibromatosis and cystic fibrosis. Other commonly inherited illnesses are either through dominant genes (when transferred directly to the descendant) or by recessive genes (when recessive genes in the genetic material from both parents are encountered) are type 2 diabetes and various cancers.

The specific tests for risk assessment to get Alzheimer's disease refer to the existence in the genome (all the genes) of genes of an individual, which are commonly associated with Alzheimer's disease or cause some changes in the brain considered responsible for the "Alzheimer's" pathology.

The role of APOE gene is well known (see the structure of different types in Appendix 4) from the somatic chromosome 19 which provides information for the synthesis of a protein called apolipoprotein E. This protein, in combination with lipids forms molecules called lipoproteins, their main role being to carry cholesterol in the blood.

The presence of the APOE gene, in form of the APOE ε4ε4 genotype determines the appearance of the extracellular amyloid deposits at affected neurons in late-onset Alzheimer dementia. Amyloidosis is even present in the early stage of the Alzheimer's disease and can be expressed by various imaging methods (see Questions 59 and 60). The analysis is performed to highlight the ε4 APOE genotype, which is a risk factor (increasing the risk of illness more than 3 times) unlike ε2 which is protective and ε3 allele which appears to be neutral.

It is to be noted that not all people who have Alzheimer dementia have the ε4 genotype, nor does the presence of this genotype (currently at 20% of the population) necessarily determine the occurrence of Alzheimer's disease.

For early-onset Alzheimer dementia (under the age of 65) there are other three specific genes: APP, PSEN 1 and PSEN2. Mutations in these genes cause excess production of toxic fragments of proteins that are grouped in extracellular β-amyloid plaques and intracellular agglomerations (neurofibrillary tangles) of modified (hyperphosphorylated) tau protein. Both are involved in the "poisoning" of neurons and their subsequent death.

Research continues on other genes that seem to have a role in dementia syndromes (not only Alzheimer's disease).

On the other hand, there are some mutagenic factors which may cause genetic mutations, among which the most active are: solar radiation, chemicals (tars from cigarettes) and single-celled living organisms which are integrated into the human DNA structure (such as viruses).

20. How common is Alzheimer's disease? How about dementia in general?

According to the latest statistics conducted in the USA (American Association Alzheimer Report 2014), the prevalence of Alzheimer's disease is one out of nine people in the population aged over 65 years. In other words, more than five million Americans suffer from dementia, with a share of over 30% for the population over 75 years.

The World Health Report 2012 "Dementia: a public health priority" has estimated that there were over 35 million people suffering from Alzheimer's disease worldwide. Due to increasing life expectancy, the Report estimates that the number will double in 2030 and will triple by 2050.

If one refers to the general population, the prevalence is about 1%, which means that in Romania (where there is no study of the current prevalence of the illness) there are approximately 200,000 people with either non-manifest (pre-dementia) or manifest Alzheimer's disease.

Other studies on the prevalence of the illness reveal the following statistics :

• Early onset DA

    40/100,000 (40-65 years onset age),

• Familial DA - early onset

    5/100,000 (genetic inheritance, the same age, 40-65

    years),

- late-onset DA

5,000/100,000 (age of onset of dementia > 65 years).

21. Is the frequency of this disease higher in more developed countries?

Basically, the frequency of the illness depends on different living standards in developed countries and the developing or poor countries. This is shown by lifestyle, diet, education but also by health assessment (or illness) in those countries.

Thus, the illness is more commonly diagnosed in developed countries due to more advanced evaluation methods (biomarkers, imaging tests). On the other hand, there are differences among developed countries mainly due to lifestyle (level of physical activity, alcohol and tobacco consumption) and especially to diet.

Thus, countries, where the "Mediterranean type" nutrition is present have a lower frequency of the illness at younger age; the same situation is encountered in countries with high consumption of fish or certain spices that are frequently used (curry, cinnamon).

22. Are there any differences between different races in the frequency of Alzheimer's disease?

Data provided by the American Alzheimer Association shows that the risk of black people to develop Alzheimer's disease is two times higher than in white population, and Hispanic population has a rate of 1.5 higher than the Caucasian population. One reason could be the presence of risk genes for Alzheimer, which are different in African-American and Hispanic population, as shown by some recent genetic studies. Another cause could be that illnesses such as hypertension and diabetes, known as vascular risk factors for Alzheimer dementia are more common in African Americans and Hispanic (this correlation would demonstrate, in a way, the role of these risk factors in the pathogenesis of Alzheimer's disease).

23. Can Alzheimer's disease be prevented? What about Alzheimer dementia?

The prevention of Alzheimer's disease also clearly includes prevention of Alzheimer dementia, the latter being the final stage of the first.

There are many ongoing studies worldwide related to prevention of Alzheimer's illness.

To be relevant, they should use subjects who "are at risk" of becoming ill from this disease (people with specific hereditary genes), but who do not have (yet) the illness' stigmata, as revealed by specific tests for Alzheimer's disease (imaging and cerebrospinal fluid examinations, less blood tests). Thus, the age at which to begin these studies should be 40 years at most, and in order for these studies to be relevant, their duration should be over 20 years and, of course, be carried out on a statistically valid number of patients, ideally in a meta-analysis (analysis made on the basis of combining the results of several studies on a large number of patients) crossborder and even across continents.

One such clinical trial (Dian study) ongoing since 2009, conducted under the coordination of the eight major US universities, assesses volunteers over 21 years who show the specific genetic profile of early onset of Alzheimer dementia (APP genes, PSEN1 and PSEN2), β antibodies action – on reducing amyloid accumulation in the brain through its regular monitoring by neuroimaging (brain metabolism - initial activity functional imaging – and subsequent structural imaging which tracks the presence or evolution of regional brain atrophy).

Similarly, the American Alzheimer's Association currently supports studies evaluating the influence of exercise, diet, cognitive and social stimulation, but also other factors considered in this illness prevention.

24. What are the structural changes in the brain in dementia?

In Alzheimer dementia, the structural macroscopic aspect (visible with the naked eye) is the cerebral atrophy. From the onset, it must be said that this criterion was excluded from the caracteristics of the Alzheimer dementia diagnostics, because in some cases, categorized as Alzheimer's, its absence has been proven (most likely rare, or other types of dementia) also, even with brain atrophy unaccompanied by dementia (maybe possible pre-dementia stages of Alzheimer's disease). Certain areas of the brain are affected more quickly in different types of dementia (Alzheimer's, fronto-temporal).

On the other hand, the medial temporal lobe atrophy measured by volumetric magnetic resonance has been reported by Leon and separately by Jack, as present in mild cognitive impairment and Alzheimer's pre-dementia.

In Viser's studies, mild atrophy was regarded as a better predictor than memory disorders (being basically a factor which can be physically observed by the doctor).

In another study, Jack considers the atrophy of medial temporal lobe as a factor independent of memory, apo-E genotype and MMSE score (an assessment of the cognitive state of a psychological type) for Alzheimer dementia. The parahippocampal gyrus volume and hippocampal volume have been pursued, the latter proving to be a more accurate risk factor between the two (brain structures involved in cognitive processes - Appendix 1).

At a cellular level, Alzheimer's dementia is characterized by:

- the presence of amyloid plaques;

- the existence of neurofibrillary deposits;

- sometimes the presence of Lewy bodies (in familial types);

- the exaggerated reactivity of the central nervous system expressed especially through the activation of the microglia (the nervous cell of support of the neuron).

The pathogenesis of Alzheimer's disease is complex because there are involved genetic factors, free radicals, citokines, neurotoxins, all having contributed beforehand to the onset of a pathogenic cascade that is still mysterious, unclear.

In vascular dementia there appear detectable modifications (computerized tomography and, even better, nuclear magnetic resonance) of ischemia secondary to stroke or indious mini-infactions (apparently asymptomatic) that occured throughout time.

25. What are the risk factors for dementias?

At this time, due to the progress of research and clinical epidemiology, the following risk factors are considered more or less important:

- Heredity (the presence of inherited specific genes) (see Question 18).
- Age - risk increases with age (over 30% for the 75 years age group).

- The presence of head trauma (including playing direct contact sports, such as rugby, American football and boxing that cause so-called pugilistic dementia or chronic traumatic encephalopathy).
- Stress - perhaps by triggering neurohormonal mechanisms.
- Vascular risk factors:

- hypertension (see Question 27);

- hypercholesterolemia (see Question 31);

- diabetes (see Question 26);

- atrial fibrillation;

- obesity;

- smoking (see Question 28).

If the two former factors can not be influenced, the latter 3 may be subject to protective or curative measures (detailed in the following questions).

Subsequent to studies in the last 10-15 years, decreased levels of vitamin B12 and folic acid are considered to be risk factors and, whether linked or not to homocysteine levels in the blood increase, hypothyroidism, lowering omega-3 unsaturated fatty acids or exposure to heavy metals.

26. Is diabetes a risk factor in Alzheimer dementia?

Diabetes (mellitus) is considered one of the key factors of vascular risk, especially in silent mode, where it "works" to impair cerebral vessels and especially small vessels. It has long been known that one of the chronic complications of diabetes is the arteriopathy in which both large and small caliber vessels are affected (macro- and micro- diabetic angiopathy). Thus, diabetes has been known to occur in myocardial infarction (silent mode), and so can the impairment of the cerebral arterioles, as well as brain microinfarctions at this level, which is equally insidious and asymptomatic.

On the other hand, recent studies show that imbalances in the insulin-glucose equilibrium cause neuronal toxicities which can damage the cognitive function more or less rapidly.

Another special situation, quite commonly seen in the geriatric practice is *the uncontrolled administration of large quantities of oral antidiabetics which can cause hypoglycemic states that are at least as toxic to neurons as hyperglycemic states.*

Once dementia is installed, frequently correlated with the occurrence of malnutrition syndrome, the weight loss determines reactivation of insulin receptor by lowering secondary glycemia, while maintaining the same dose of antidiabetic agents (whether oral or different types of insulin administered subcutaneously). That's why I recommend a frequent glycemic control (having a daily schedule - morning, noon, evening and night) to adjust the dosage of antidiabetics and prevent hypoglycemic states.

On the other hand, oral antidiabetic drug doses must be constantly adjusted considering the decline of renal function in the elderly, their replacement with human insulin preparations being most useful.

27. *Is hypertension a risk factor in dementia?*

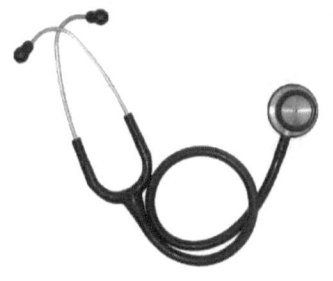

Hypertension (essential or secondary) is by its high frequency in the geriatric population (over 60% except

Asians and northern peoples - including Iceland), the most important vascular risk factor. On the other hand, it is and can most easily be controllable by antihypertensive medication and adequate sodium diet (low sodium).

Injuries that are brought upon the endothelium (internal area of the blood vessel) by the sudden increase in blood pressure, are initially presented in the form of micro-cracks, followed by local micro-hemorrhages and then by a repair reaction through forming a micro-thrombus which may partially obstruct the blood vessel and then, over time, completely causing death of the cells (neurons, microglia, etc.) served by the respective vessel. The impact on small vessels is associated at autopsy especially with vascular dementia, but can also appear in Alzheimer dementia.

That is why blood pressure control is vital for prevention of neurodegenerative illnesses, the maintenance of 120-130 mmHg values for systolic blood pressure ("the large one") and under 80 mmHg for diastolic blood pressure ("the small one"), are considered optimal. Monitoring must be carried out in the morning and evening and whenever the subject shows specific symptoms (headache, dizziness, tinnitus – noise in the ears, or worse, nausea and vomiting in hypertensive encephalopathy).

28. Is smoking a risk factor in dementia?

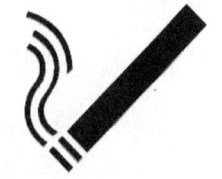

Absolutely yes. There is no secret that smoking is harmful both for consumers and for the passive smokers. It is a major risk factor for cancer and cardiovascular illnesses.

A WHO report in 2014 attributed smoking to 14% of cases of Alzheimer dementia worldwide.

But what would the mechanisms be by which the tobacco is involved in determining or influencing memory illnesses? On one hand smoking accelerates the process of atherosclerosis – aging blood vessels, a process which begins since the embryonic stage of the individual! - And on the other hand, it increases plasma levels of homocysteine, an independent risk factor for stroke and, more recently, for Alzheimer dementia.

A third course of action is considered to increase the cellular oxidative stress associated with excitotoxicity associated with smoking, which eventually leads to neuron death and damage following specific neurocognitive dementias.

29. Is there any relationship between stress and dementia?

There are many ongoing studies on the action of stress (particularly "chronic stress") as a risk factor in dementia. Some studies in mice have shown that high levels of chronic stress can cause damage in the hippocampus and induce impaired short-term memory. The mechanism involved is determined by increased blood glucose (in fact, blood sugar imbalances) and secondarily by the increased stress hormones – corticosteroids.

Another recent study showed that constant increased levels of cortisol cause gradual loss of synapses in the prefrontal cortex (associated with short-term memory). According to this study, cortisol has a "corrosive" action directly on the synapses. The researchers suggest that there could be benefits from normalization of cortisol in patients with traumatic or chronic stress.

30. Are people with more education more prone to Alzheimer dementia?

Studies on this topic are still contradictory, although the consensus is that a high degree of education is an important preventive factor in dementia, if not at least to delay its appearance.

Until recently (including in the context of earlier studies ("The Nun study"), it has been considered that all the means of "cognitive stimulation" (see Questions 41-43) delay the onset of cognitive deterioration process so that more educated people would suffer less likely from dementia than those less educated.

On the other hand, a recent study raises the possibility that excessive neuronal stimulation (likely associated with chronic stress) determines the toxicity secondary to increased oxidative stress which ultimately leads to neuronal death and subsequently to dementia.

31. Can high cholesterol in the blood cause Alzheimer's disease?

As it has been known for a long time, after some meta-analysis (including the Framingham study) blood cholesterol is of two types: the good, which protects from stroke - HDL cholesterol and the bad - LDL cholesterol that helps form plaque, and it is involved in obstruction of blood vessels and secondarily in the appearance of strokes with different locations (heart - the coronary arteries or brain common carotid artery and/or internal and cerebral arteries) but also in small and very small blood vessels, as specific in Alzheimer dementia and in some vascular or mixed dementia.

If these pathological processes are only a risk factor or trigger the "Alzheimer's", pathology remains to be determined in future research.

32. Can thyroid disease cause a form of dementia?

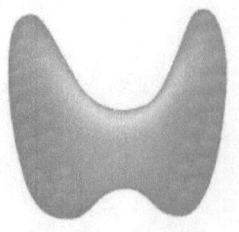

Thyroid illnesses are mainly caused by iodine deficiency in the diet as a phenomenon of population/area (so-called "goatee zones" - one third of the world population living in these areas). Also, there is a hypothyroidism induced by a total thyroidectomy used as a means in radical treatment of some thyroid tumors or other pathological conditions of the thyroid.

The specialty literature discusses the connection between hypothyroidism and cognitive impairment, up to severe impairment of cognition and daily activities and causing so-called "thyroid dementia." The relationship seems logical considering that the thyroid, since the growth period, has a role in shaping the nervous system (thyroid hormone deficiency in childhood leading to an illness that is increasingly rare, called cretinism).

Despite long time knowledge of this type of dementia, it is characterized by underdiagnosis. Too fast and without being well investigated, dementia syndromes are diagnosed as "Alzheimer's" or, more recently, as "mixed". The situation is especially sad because diagnosis, or even suspicion thereof, can be quickly set by an ordinary dosing of blood markers of thyroid function (T3, T4 - TSH and thyroid hormone - pituitary hormonal regulator of T3 and T4). And more importantly, early diagnosis of this correlation - thyroid dysfunction/dementia – would cause partial or total cognitive impairment reversal, thyroid dementia being part of reversible dementias class (see Question 56).

There is a debate at what level of TSH hypothyroidism must be considered, bearing in mind that currently, values between 0.5-5 are accepted as normal. A recent study showed a statistically valid correlation between a TSH greater than 2.1 and the risk of developing dementia (Alzheimer dementia is the correlation of this study). The increased frequency of both thyroid dysfunction (4 of 5) and Alzheimer dementia (2 of 3 – American Alzheimer's Association Report 2014) reported among women in the general population are consistent with this hypothesis.

33. Can heart disease cause dementia?

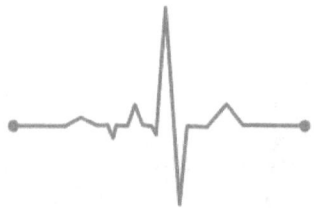

I wrote earlier about the involvement of hypertension as a risk factor in the pathology of vascular dementias (see Question 27). A tighter control of hypertension lowers the risk of vascular damage, but due to changes on the blood vessels with age (baroreceptors role in regulating blood pressure), one should make a careful verification of the dynamics of blood pressure, and evaluate the need of decreasing dosage in antihypertensive medication in order not to cause hypotension and secondary to it, a cerebral hypoperfusion which ultimately leads to a deficit of the cerebral functions (not just cognition). The hypotension may also cause falls and their complications (most commonly and severely being a femur fracture).

Another heart illness which correlates with dementia is atrial fibrillation; in this case, at least two mechanisms are involved. The first and most important is the increased risk of sending small fragments of thrombus (blood clot) located in the left atrium. These fragments can be localized at the level of small blood vessels in the brain obstructing them and causing downstream ischemia (irrigated neurons by these blood vessels). The second mechanism could be that within the atrial fibrillation, 30% of the pumping function of the heart is lost by ineffective flashing contractions (almost imperceptible) of the atria, as the brain is dependent on a large amount of blood sent from the heart (25% of the blood flow reaches the brain).

Another situation I recently came across in two cases, is the heart pacemaker failure with setting-in of bradycardia or even cardiac arrest. Considering that these are usually patients with severe heart conditions and reduced functional reserve (see Question 39), the conditions are met for the transformation of a medium undiagnosed cognitive impairment in a form ranging from mild to severe dementia, directly proportional to the length of brain hypoxia secondary to the cardiac event.

34. What is mild cognitive impairment? What about subjective cognitive impairment?

Mild cognitive impairment is a syndrome characterized by intellectual deterioration - in which recent memory impairment is the most common, possibly but not necessarily, the only one – not severe enough to affect one's daily activities.

Over time, more than half of the patients progress into a form of dementia. Thus, the main role of the research in the field is to increase predictability of evolution into dementia, such as to allow the introduction of pharmacological therapies which delay or even stop the emergence of dementia.

Mild Cognitive Impairment (MCI) is a nonspecific term and is imperfect as it encourages generalization for a wide variety of cognitive disorders. MCI can be diagnosed if a patient has normal cognitive functions but no dementia (PJVisser, 2005).

Mild cognitive impairment can be "pure" or "impure".

- **Pure MCI** - mild cognitive impairment which will not develop into dementia, considered equivalent with benign brain aging

- **Impure MCI** – mild cognitive impairment which will develop into dementia in some indefinite time

In the specialty literature, the impure MCI is called the prodromal phase of Alzheimer dementia (90% of MCI turns Alzheimer dementia, although it can precede other forms of dementia too).

At this time, the delimitation pure/impure MCI is only retrospectively possible (after developing dementia).

The mild cognitive impairment has several forms, depending on the type of cognitive dysfunction involved (amnestic or non-amnestic amnesia form, monodomain/multiple domains). Although there is no reliable correlation, identification of the clinical form for mild cognitive disorder is important as a prognostic factor of the form of dementia toward which it may progress (Alzheimer dementia, vascular dementia, dementia associated with Parkinson's disease, diffuse Lewy body illness, frontotemporal dementia, etc.).

Diagnostic criteria for mild cognitive impairment have been shaped and then improved around 2000 by the great professor of neurology R.C. Petersen.

1999

• Memory disorders reported by the patient, family and physician

• Normal daily activity (ADL - normal)

• Normal global cognitive function

• Clinical dementia rating of 0.5

• Objective Memory Disorders.

• Non-demented patient (per DSM IV criteria).

2001

- Impaired memory preferably evidenced by others.

- Memory Disorders measurable by standardized tests.

- Normal thinking and judgment.

- Normal daily activity (ADL - normal).

- Non-demented patient (per DSM IV criteria).

There are other diagnostic criteria but those formulated by Petersen are today widely regarded as the most well structured.

The yearly conversion rate to dementia:

- **MCI: 12-13%**.
    - Normal patient (without obvious cognitive impairment) only **1%**.

This rate varies significantly from one study to another.

Visser & Bruscoli's meta-analysis are the most credible, showing that the annual conversion rate is 10% and is limited to 50% of the subjects.

The early diagnosis, even from this phase, would provide immediate benefits both to the patient and the society from an economical standpoint.

> **Nota bene!**
>
> One has to differentiate between the mild cognitive impairment – which is equivalent to the mild cognitive deficit, and the minor neurocognitive disorders (DSM V classification) – which is equivalent to mild cognitive impairment and mild dementia.

An even newer concept than the mild cognitive impairment is the subjective cognitive deterioration which would precede it as part of the Alzheimer's illness, and which corresponds with the preclinical phase timewise, and which – until recently – has been considered asymptomatic (Thus, it precedes the Alzeimer's illness onset by 15-20 years.).

This subjective cognitive deterioration can only be recognized by the patient (the psychometric tests for cognition are perfect!) who talks about a "memory weakening" and some cognition-related phenomena becoming worrisome to them;

have difficulties orienting themselves in new locations, forget where they placed their car keys, or the paragraphs in the book they were reading, to start again the next day…

The subjective cognitive deterioration may be an alarm signal for the involved person to adopt a healty diet (e.g. the Mediterranean diet), and exclude some vices and excesses in their life. Likewise, they can work with a memory illness specialist for an appropriate tracking of their evolution over the years and decades to come.

35. How can we find out whether the mild cognitive impairment precedes dementia?

Early stages of Alzheimer's illness are:

- **preclinical phase** - Alzheimer's illness, an asymptomatic period;

- **prodromal phase** - Alzheimer's illness, mild cognitive impairment stage;

• **early diagnostic phase** - diagnostic criteria for dementia are met.

Possible pathophysiological evolution scheme in cognitive disorders can be identified in Appendix 5.

Distinguishing subjects with mild disorders of cognition who will develop dementia from those with mild cognitive deficiency from other causes, such as depression and normal aging, is a major clinical problem. At the present time, there is no way/algorhythm to differentiate these types of early deterioration of intellectual functions.

36. What are the biomarkers of Alzheimer's disease? Where and when do they occur?

Due to the increasing incidence of dementia in general and Alzheimer dementia in particular, criteria are required for early diagnosis even from mild cognitive impairment stage, – it would be ideal if possible – in the preclinical phase of dementia. In order to achieve an early diagnosis, specific cognitive tests, laboratory tests (MRI hippocampus, SPECT, PET – photon emission computed tomography), but also laboratory analysis for the determination of specific substances for this illness, known as humoral biomarkers or biomarkers are being used.

A study of clinical data correlated with SPECT performed on a group of 70 patients showed an increase in the dignostics degree of association of both diagnostic methods (92% versus 84% in terms of using clinical data alone).

By definition, biological markers (biomarkers) can reflect a variety of illnesses including specific level of exposure to environmental factors and genetic illness, specific substance (possibly in an intermediate stage between exposure and onset of illness) or an independent factor associated with a stage of the illness.

Depending on the specific characteristics of biomarkers, they can be used to identify the illness risk (precursor biomarkers), identification of illness (diagnostics biomarkers) or predictive of illness stages, including response to therapy (prognostic biomarkers).

Optimal use of biomarkers should be made easily and quickly and be cost effective, safe for both the patient and physician, and possess sensitivity, specificity and predictive value, of course.

Other proposed criteria for Alzheimer's biomarkers:

1. The ideal biomarkers for cognitive impairment and dementia should easily detect the basic criteria of the illness' neuropathology.

2. The testing should be noninvasive, easy to be performed and inexpensive.

3. Only those biomarkers which have beneficial effects should be used, possibly in the change of treatment.

4. Identification of antecedent biomarkers of Alzheimer dementia is a very important goal (precursor biomarkers are those that can be found in the phase of mild cognitive impairment or Alzheimer predementia).

5. Ideally, the precursor biomarkers should have an essential feature: the ability to detect pathology in the preclinical stage. Because the pathogenesis of Alzheimer's begins many years before the symptoms of the illness, their study implies supporting or even suspecting a preclinical diagnosis.

6. The precursor (preclinical) biomarkers are useful not only in screening and diagnosis of the illness but also in identifying the target population for new antidemential drugs.

7. They also may serve as a target for new prophylactic therapies and possibly as a starting point in testing the efficacy of new drugs in the research stage.

Biomarkers may be classified into:

• **Genetic Biomarkers** identified through genomic studies (see Questions 18 and 19):

- "genomics",

- "proteomics".

• **CSF Biomarkers:**

- beta – amyloid,

- tau protein,

- isoprostans,

- sulphatides.

• **Neuroimaging Biomarkers:**

- structural and metabolic changes in the structural and functional imaging.

CSF Biomarkers:

Predictive:

Low extracellular β-amyloid levels.

Increased intracellular level of tau protein.

Increased intracellular level of hyperphosphorylated tau protein.

Probably higher accuracy of diagnostic for combination increased Tau protein/decreased amyloid beta combination.

The beta – amyloid:

Slow buildup of plaques containing the extracellular amyloid beta is characteristic of Alzheimer dementia. Aß peptides of 40-43 amino acids long (Aß 1-40, Aß 1-42, Aß 1-43) are normal by-products derived from an amyloid precursor protein (APP) through a proteolytic process.

An overproduction occurs in AD, the fragments of Aß 1-40 increasing and/or Aß oligomers 1-42 which gather

forming insoluble oligomers as a result of genetic changes (see Question 19). Insoluble peptides agglomerate and together with neuronal degradation products form plaques observed in AD. The aggregation of Aß in the brain occur years (if not decades) before specific symptoms of AD.

However, post-mortem detection of amyloid plaque formation can not be used as a biomarker, but only to confirm the diagnosis.

This beta-amyloid deposits can be identified by measuring specific parameters of CSF and brain interstitial fluid, mos recently by microdialysis. CSF Aβ42 levels in Alzheimer dementia is significantly decreased compared with the witness group, but there are differences between studies. The level is also significantly decreased in slight cognitive impairment as compared to the control group.

Highlighting blood Aß is possible but nonspecific (also present in renal diseases).

Because of the Aß accumulation in the brain since the preclinical stage of Alzheimer's disease, theoretically, the Aß candidate is "the most important biomarker" in both the preclinical diagnosis (as precursor biomarker) and the postclinical diagnosis (as a diagnostic biomarker). However, its identification is not specific to be used alone (i.e. not pathognomonic).

Along with the understanding of the the metabolism and the elimination of Aß in plasma, using the measurement of its level in blood is likely to increase (because the half-time of Aß in the blood is very short – approximately 10-15 minutes).

The tau protein is essential for the diagnosis of dementia in certain pathological conditions and is present in:

• Neurofibrillary tangles,

• Neuropil networks,

• Neuritic plaques.

The neuronal cytoskeleton is composed of neurofilaments and microtubules (with an important role in the transport of substances with a nutritional role within the neuron) being essential for normal neuronal function and for making the connection between the neuronal synapse and body. The neurofibrillary balls located intraneurally are composed of helical pairs of filaments composed of tau protein aggregates.

The neurofibrillary degeneration consists of some dense fiber fascicles arranged as some balls inside the neurons, mainly composed of tau protein that suffers an abnormal process of hyperphosphorylation.

Isoprostans: Isomers of prostaglandin produced by oxidative modification of PUFA (polyunsaturated fatty acids) by a mecanism catalyzed by free radicals (recently regarded as biomarkers of Alzheimer's).

Prostaglandins play an important part in various physiological and pathological processes (hormonal regulation, functioning of the sympathetic nervous system, the mechanism of inflammation, smooth muscle contraction) and can be used in the treatment of gastrointestinal ulcers.

The isoprostans accumulate in tissues, circulating in plasma and are excreted in urine. F2-IPS (isoprostan CNS) is a specific biomarker for Alzheimer dementia in conditions of increasing its concentration in the cerebrospinal fluid, blood or urine.

The oxidative stress in the central nervous system is manifested predominantly as lipid peroxidation. The process of lipid peroxidation was traditionally linked to poor specificity/sensitivity for Alzheimer dementia. It is unclear whether lipid peroxidation is a consequence of the neurodegenerative process or the two processes are independent.

There are currently known precursor biomarkers, diagnostic markers, but there are not known "pathognomonic" markers in Alzheimer dementia. By using the determinations of these biomarkers in combination, their specificity and sensitivity increase.

Biomarkers – those known and others which remain to be discovered in the future – probably remain crucial in the diagnosis of Alzheimer in preclinical stage.

37. Why is the early diagnosis of Alzheimer's disease important?

Early recognition of a progressive degenerative dementia offers patients the opportunity to express or clarify their life plans while their judgment and personality are still intact and allow families to start planning the financial aspects for the care of the affected person.

It is estimated that over 25 million people worldwide have dementia, with 4.6 million new cases of dementia each year (one new case every 7 seconds). The number of the affected people will double every 20 years to reach 81.1 million by 2040. In 2014, the United States spent over 220 billion dollars to treat this condition.

An early diagnosis of the illness would extend the phases considered as lighter (mild cognitive impairment, dementia in mild and medium phases), which are less expensive and would shorten the final phase (severe dementia) characterized by bed confinement and its complications (lung or urinary infections, brain or heart strokes, bedsores), thus involving costs 8-10 times higher than in mild stages. A simple calculation shows that the delay of non-invalidating dementia phases by only five years, would halve the number of patients with this pathology, which would mean halving huge amounts spent by both the community and by the families.

On the other hand, early recognition of reversible dementia (see Question 56) may lead to its cure, with all positive implications at the individual and community level. There has been limited interest in the extended, differential diagnosis beyond exclusion of the "traditional" reversible dementias.

38. Can we improve our memory?

The cerebral cortex is composed of a hundred billion neurons, connected by a network of logic axonal circuits of 175,000 km with all brain structures. The neuron is the structural and functional unit cell of the nervous system and the body is made up of neurons and its extensions (axons and dendrites) required to make up the synapses (connections) between neurons. Between axons there are 60,000 billion short and long term synapses (gaps). They act like small semiconductor diodes (40 nm), which transmit current at low voltages (unidirectional transmission), at a high communication speed (240 km/h). 250,000 neurons are connected per minute with other neurons, contributing to the formation of a neural network which can be likened to a spider web. The development of each new structure (and function), complements the previous one, showing the potential of "regeneration" of the nervous system.

Memory is one of the complex cognitive functions, required for storing the information learned throughout life, resulting in permanent mental processes (including during sleep, in the REM phase). The learning process involves three ways: visual, auditive and semantic, but the information selection has also an emotional support. Memory implies complex processing: Attention - Information Capture - Encoding - Storing - Decoding - Playing. The information flow is similar to a computer. The best method is the visual memory and even visual and spatial (visual and spatial correlation of the characteristics of objects). According to some authors this type of memory is affected first in Alzheimer dementia.

Memory classification may be accomplished depending either on the time and duration (anterograde, retrograde, short or long) or the mode of action (working memory, semantic memory, episodic or procedural). The most affected of all is episodic memory, lasting minutes to years, whereby the patient can not access the newly learned information, has trouble concentrating but can erroneously correlate different information received.

Permanent stimulation of the complex cognitive functions, including storing, leading to "settling" of branch lines (synapses and neurotransmitters from synapses) between different neural structures making them durable and sustainable, increasing the cognitive functional reserve (see Question 39).

The mind, responsible for the mental processes, is the result of ceaseless activity of the brain. Everything that has been accomplished by homo sapiens (modern man) was originally represented in his mind.

It is said that **"A permanently trained brain never gets tired!"** just as **"If you do not use it, you lose it!"**

39. What is cognitive reserve?

Cognitive reserve represents the degree of functional compensation of a cognitive impairment. In my opinion, "cognitive frailty" is present in the older people without dementia but also in the different types of dementia. In other words, there is a functional cognitive reserve (lower, of course) which can be used, exploited on patients with established dementia. To include both situations, we propose a new entity called "Cognitive frailty syndrome in older people with or without dementia".

The annual report of the International Alzheimer's Association 2014 "Alzheimer's Disease – Facts and Figures" highlights that a greater number of years of education build up a cognitive reserve able to better compensate changes due to the existence of a minor or major neurocognitive disorder (DSM V - Appendix 2).

The role of cognitive growth reserve: the increase of cognitive reserve and preserving it would delay the 6 and 7 Reisberg stages (the terminal stages of dementia) and shorten them. As I said, shortening the disabling phases of dementia determines benefits at both the individual and population level (economic).

> Cognitive reserve hypothesis shows that increased educational level increases the number of synapses between neurons, neuronal machinery to compensate for changes in Alzheimer's disease through the use of "alternate neuron-to-neuron communication routes".

The phenomenon mechanism is similar to the ischemic heart illness occurring at middle age in which there is a collateral circulation through new vessels derived from the coronary arteries, which prevents the occurrence of acute myocardial infarction.

Some researchers believe that the risk of dementia among people with low educational level can be explained by other factors, such as common low socioeconomic level and low access to the health care system.

In the same way, the concept of cognitive health came along, which depends on a number of protective factors, as well as risk factors which influence the neurocognitive activity (the term mental health is a term too broad including other areas of brain activity). This concept is very useful for educating people in the prevention of cognitive pathology.

40. Is there a cognitive frailty syndrome of the elderly?

In general, the frailty syndrome, is said to be a concept that one can not define but immediately recognize when one sees it. It is equivalent to the risk of severe morbidity or diminished healing ability. The cognitive frailty syndrome can be defined similarly.

The relationship "cognitive frailty" – "cognitive reserve" is obviously inversely proportional: a diminished cognitive reserve determines an increased cognitive frailty and of course vice versa, a high cognitive reserve determines a much lower cognitive frailty syndrome.

An international meeting organized by the International Academy on Nutrition and Aging (IANA) and Association of Gerontology and Geriatrics International (IAGG) held in Toulouse in 2013 describes an International Consensus Group on "Cognitive frailty". The final report contains the results of the consensus group and provides the first definition of "Cognitive frailty in older adults". The main purpose of this first approach was to facilitate the achievement of a specific framework for a personalized prevention intervention on the elderly, in this area.

The consensus group proposes to identify the so-called "cognitive frailty" as a heterogeneous group of clinical manifestations characterized by the simultaneous presence of physical frailty and cognitive impairment, which will sooner or later ultimately lead to expression of the dementia syndrome.

In particular, key factors to define "cognitive frailty" as they were proposed by that group of consensus include:

1. The presence of physical frailty and cognitive disorder (Clinical Dementia Rating scale, CDR = 0.5);

2. Exclusion of this Alzheimer dementia and other types of dementia.

A potential reversibility may characterize this entity.

The psychopathological component of this condition is obvious and participates in the increased vulnerability of the body to individual stressors.

In various circumstances, cognitive fragility may be a precursor of neurodegenerative processes.

Finally, the group discusses the use of an intervention focused on the physical, nutritional, cognitive and psychological domains, in order to improve the quality of life in elderly people with cognitive frailty or risk.

41. What is cognitive stimulation?

Cognitive stimulation (or therapy of cognitive stimulation TCS) is the set of activities through which the intellectual – cognitive capabilities of an individual are hightlighted and activated, having as main purpose to improve mental performance by increasing cognitive reserve and implicitly preventing memory illnesses.

COGNITION *noun.* The faculty of knowing or the process by which understanding is developed in the mind (< Fr. Cognition, lat. Cognitio).

The roles of cognitive stimulation:

• Improvement of the cognitive status, of abstract and conceptual thinking, of language

• Improvement of the behavioral disorders and decrease of the degree of depression

• Increase of social networking

• Improvement of skills needed in daily activities

Brief history:

The psychological type therapy in dementia (as the temporal-spatial orientation) has been used by nearly half a century. Despite its longevity, the effects remain questionable because, unfortunately, many of these studies were either short or poor as methodology.

Temporospatial orientation operates by presenting and repeating the guidance information either throughout the day

("24 hours") or in groups engaged in orientation activities ("Class").

One study has established that the orientation has been associated with significant improvements in both cognition and behavior, but identified the need for large, multi-centric, well-organized trials.

The results of this study were used to develop a therapy program focused on cognitive stimulation.

Cognitive stimulation is done through various exercises (described below) which appeal to emotional (affective) stimulation. The affective stimulation is the set of tools used to restore a mentally balanced status, resistant to stress factors on a patient with dementia accompanied by depressive and behavioral disorders, regardless of the stage of the illness, except for the severe ones (Stage 6, 7 of the Reisberg scale).

The roles of emotional stimulation are:

• Regaining self-confidence

• Reducing anxiety, depression

• Improving communication and social reintegration

42. What are the simplest cognitive stimulation exercises?

The cognitive stimulation, as we have seen its definition (see the previous question), is carried out through any activity which triggers the intellectual functions and particularly the cognitive activity. These should be correlated to cognitive impairment, starting from more complex exercises in the stage of mild cognitive impairment and getting to the easiest in advanced stages of dementia.

Below are some easy exercises that anyone can solve at home:

In the mild cognitive disorder:

• Games which stimulate thinking (complex cognitive functions): chess, crosswords, canasta, bridge, sudoku

• Remembering a time, in writing, with as many details of a movie seen before (the description of the place and time, of the characters, the emotions experienced during the movie, etc.). It is advisable to watch movies on the weekends, i.e. on a Saturday night, and remembering to do the exercise the next morning. The evaluation of such exercises is done by a psychologist, but even without the evaluation, this exercise is useful when carried out systematically.

• Writing essays or poems, then analysing them

In the constituted cognitive disorder:

• Daily temporospatial orientation exercices

• Exercises of identification and naming of proper names, names of family members, colleagues, friends

• Exercises for object identification, their color

• Exercises of verbal fluency (the patient is asked to voice in a fixed period – 1 or 2 minutes – as many words from a semantic group or as many words which begin with a specific letter).

• Learning some new songs

• Stimulation of unactivated hobbies (painting, group reading or singing, gardening when time and health status of the patient allow)

Some examples of simple exercices:

- Poems in the "magic hat": in a bowl, place tickets with the titles of some 3 stanzas/4 lyrics poems. Participants extract single tickets and are asked to read the poem aloud. At the end of the program the participants will be asked to recite as many verses from the chosen poetry.
- Recognition of famous characters: Shows one photo representing a famous character to each participant. Participants must recognize the chosen character. Group discussions are then carried out about that character.
- The backpack filled with items for a trip: images of things, some of which are needed are being displayed. Participants must choose the items needed for the trip and place them in the backpack.
- Conversation Lesson: groups of 2-3 people are being formed. Participants are engaged in a free discussion.
- Card Game selection: 5 cards are dealt to each game participant. They are asked to choose the cards representing diamonds or spades and place them face up on the table.

In recent years, a great deal of programs to stimulate intellectual functions have been developed over the Internet. On a simple search "brain exercises to improve memory", a search engine provided us with more than 42 million distinct pages, indicating a huge interest for this type of cognitive stimulation.

On the other hand, some researchers have shown that simple surfing is a great for cognitive stimulation, especially as it activates the type of complex functions, as selecting, prioritizing and analyzing different information on the same subject. This type of activity is even recommended for at least one hour per day, which would have a significant effect at the neuronal level even in patients already diagnosed with Alzheimer's.

43. Until what stage of the illness can the cognitive stimulation be used?

Cognitive stimulation can be achieved until stage 6 is also included on the Reisberg scale (severe cognitive impairment. Intermediate Alzheimer's type dementia) when cognitive functions are still maintained.

The Reisberg Scale is presented in Appendix 6.

Exercises which can be performed refer to identification and practice of greeting forms, of correct addressing formulas for expressing feelings, emotions, sentiments but also work to identify and call the proper names, names of various acquaintances (relatives, friends).

It is obvious that the last stage, 7 on the Reisberg scale, when the patient has brain activity limited only to archaic reflexes, these efforts are needless.

44. Do physical exercises help improve memory?

Lately, the role of exercise (especially aerobic) in improving cognition and its appropriate use is being studied more and more (depending on age and coexisting pathology) in patients with dementia.

To understand the mechanisms triggered in the of relation physical exercise-cognition improvement we briefly describe the two types of exercises - aerobic and anaerobic.

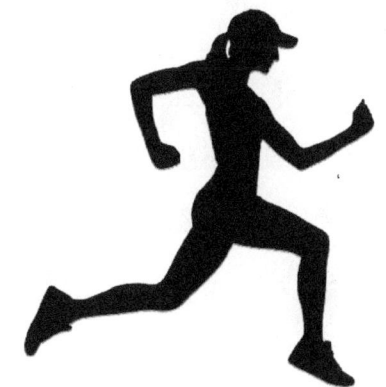

The aerobic effort occurs when muscle energy arises by burning ergogenic substances in the presence of oxygen. This category of aerobic effort includes activities that involve large muscle groups: fast walking, jogging, cycling, swimming, and rowing. They induce adaptive changes in the respiratory and circulatory system, but also at the level of various metabolic pathways. Cardio training improves the capacity of the respiratory and circulatory systems, increases blood flow, increases the ability of muscles to produce energy via aerobic means and metabolize the fat.

The anaerobic effort is the effort whereby the energy is generated by burning ergogenic substances with a lack of oxygen. The anaerobic effort can be of two types: alactacid anaerobic effort and lactacid anaerobic effort.

The lactacyd anaerobic effort

The duration of these efforts is a maximum of 60 seconds. The energy substrate based on which ATP is being re-synthesised, is represented by the carbohydrates. The glucose or glycogen are degraded inside the cell (intracytoplasmic) through anaerobiosis (chemical processes carried out without oxygen), a process called anaerobic glycolysis. The anaerobic degradation of carbohydrates is incomplete, leading to lactic acid, hence the name of lactacid effort. Examples of anaerobic efforts lactacid are running the 200m, 400m and 4x400m laps.

The A-lactacyd anaerobic effort

The energy substrate of this effort type is represented by another system: the one of phosphagenics (represented by the adenosine triphosphates – ATP and creatine kinase – CK) which, thorough the catalized reactions by the myosyin ATPase and Phosphofructokinase enzymes, explosively frees a large quantity of energy through breakage of the phosphate links. The A-lactacyd anaerobic efforts are strength and spring.

The benefits of physical exercise in humans:

• reduced cardiovascular risk,

• it increases blood flow to the brain,

• it controls blood pressure,

• it improves lipid metabolism,

• it prevents type 2 diabetes,

• weight control,

- it improves "wellness" and quality of life,

- it helps maintain bone mineral density,

- it increases fibrinolytic activity,

- it decreases inflammation,

- it improves endothelial function,

- possible antiarrhythmic effect by increasing vagal tone,

- it improves sleep quality,

- it may improve immune function,

- reducing cancer risk.

The benefits of physical exercise in patients with dementia:

- it increases cerebral blood flow,

- it slows brain atrophy (especially in parahippocampus and temporal cortex),

- some studies show a marked decrease in the rate of decline in MMSE and other cognitive tests,

- it improves the quality of life and ADL score - Activity Daily Living and IADL – Instrumental Activity Daily Living (see Appendix 7),

- it decreases the risk of falls and fractures.

Recent studies coordinated by Carl Cotman of the University of California have shown that *repeated exercises stimulate the release of a neurotrophin called BDNF (brain - derived - neurotrophic - factor) especially in the hippocampus, hub of learning and memory, which increases volume and development of new synapses of neurons. Further reinforcing the discharge of BDNF could slow cognitive decline in patients who already have specific structural changes of Alzheimer's disease.*

The physical effort should be carried out gradually according to the associated pathology and is expressed in MET units.

MET (metabolic equivalent) is the ratio of a person's metabolic rate at rest and metabolic rate of a person performing physical activity.

1 MET is equivalent to the metabolic rate of oxygen consumption of 3.5 ml of oxygen per kilogram of body weight per minute.

The Metabolic Equivalent (MET) during various activities is shown in Appendix 8.

Elderly patient exercise depending on the intensity of activity can be followed in Appendix 9.

Various exercise programs have been developed as result of these studies, especially in the United States, tailored to different types of illness, which generally recommend a time of 150 minutes weekly, in different daily modules. For example, for patients with cardiac pathology, walking is recommended in three daily sessions of 10 minutes each, 5 times weekly.

45. *What are the limits of physical exercise in dementia?*

The only limits in performing physical exercise for a patient with dementia are linked to the presence of cardiac illness and/or lung damage. And, as we know, heart illness and hypertension, atrial fibrillation, valvular heart illness may be associated with vascular dementia, so they can frequently coexist with dementias. The monitoring of blood pressure and heart rate (pulse) during physical exercise is compulsory and, in our experience with such patients, exercise should not exceed an effort 2 MET (light effort for age group) for 20-30 minutes 4-5 times per week (walking on ground level under 3 km/hour, with minimum speed gradually starting at 0.8 km/hour).

For patients without significant associated cardiac pathology, exercises can be used within the limit of 4 MET (stationary bike < 16 km/h) under the same conditions (20-30 minutes 4-5 times a week). For patients with hemiparesis and strokes, passive bike riding will be used initially to restore passive walking.

The introduction of these programs helps improve general health, resistance to infections, but also of heart and lung function, which we consider to be appropriate both in a specialized setting (hospital center for long-term care) and in the homecare of patients.

Another possibility (this time accurate) to measure daily physical activity, including for patients who can not perform dedicated daily activities (heart illnesses), is to use a pedometer, a device which measures the number of steps, a total of over 7500 daily steps being considered sufficient to fit the patient in the category of "at least moderate physical activity" sufficient to prevent (to the possible extent) cardiovascular and implicitly neurovascular illnesses, including in Alzheimer's pathology.

46. What are the costs of care in Alzheimer dementia?

The costs related to caring for a patient with dementia vary depending on the stage of the illness but also on medical and social services in the country. According to the Alzheimer's Facts and Figures report published in 2014 by the American Alzheimer's Association, in 2013 in the United States families and friends of patients with dementia conducted over 17 billion hours of care that would be worth over 220 billion dollars.

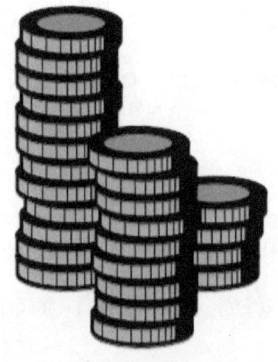

In 2014 the direct costs within the American Society for Alzheimer's illness treatment and care have reached more than 200 billion dollars.

Costs per patient at a stage where a patient must hospitalized on long-term (nursing home Long-Term Care) ranges from about $1,000/month in less developed countries (the South-East Europe) to over $3000 in the US and over $4000 in countries in northern Europe.

47. What are the stages of Alzheimer's disease? What about Alzheimer dementia?

The Alzheimer's disease stages reflect the states of Alzheimer's illness (as described in Question 8).

Regarding the stages of Alzheimer dementia – given its slow, progressive evolution - we can consider them to be intertwined, the clinical differentiation only being made by experienced specialists. There are certain scores on psychometric assessment corresponding to stages (states) for mild, moderate and severe dementia (see Question 59).

After studying more than 5,000 cases over the past 10 years, I have proposed in the Appendix 10, the following assessment of cognitive impairment and its states, starting from the verification of the activities which the person being evaluated can carry out, resulting in several stages, ranging from the stage without cognitive impairment (considered "the normal phase") up to the severe stage of the illness. Correlating my own study data with that obtained from the specialty literature, I have also established the average duration of the illness progression in those stages.

The evaluation of illness stage in the proposed schedule is performed starting on the right column (severe stage) to the left column (generally called – the normal phase - in which the pacients shows no cognitive symptomatology). The first column (taken in the order shown above) in which three clinical criteria are being met, represents the patient's disease stage at that time.

I should mention that the survival prognosis, based on that same study, is a statistical one, some patients, usually in the presence of other serious illnesses (heart illness, cancer), do not reach the average, while in other cases (special care conditions, swift action on infections, on hydro-electrolyte imbalances), patients go 1-2 years beyond these limitations.

48. Can we quickly assess the stage of the disease?

It is obvious that in the preclinical stage of Alzheimer's there are no clinical milestones to detect its presence. The only possibility is by investigating the diagnostic markers and the biomarkers of illness (see Question 36), but as they are expensive, they are only carried out in a research context.

Largely, the mild cognitive impairment (MCI - Mild Cognitive Impairment), as we defined it (see Question 34), refers to cognitive disorders more or less severe but which do not cause harm to the daily activity of the person. So, any memory disorder accompanied by alterations in specific psychometric tests should put us on guard to the possibility of a mild cognitive impairment, as a precursor of dementia (Alzheimer's or another dementia). Diagnosis can not be sustained unless a subsequent assessment reveals a worsening of cognitive impairment or even the evolution towards a constituted dementia.

Once dementia is constituted, that is, a cognitive impairment that is significant enough to change the patient's daily activity, it is just a question of determining the stage of dementia. This is done by connecting clinical data with cognitive assessment scores (see Question 59) and requires the expertise of a specialist, since this stage of the disease correlates with prognosis (see Question 47 – Appendix 7).

49. What is the first typical sign of Alzheimer's?

Obviously, the first typical sign of Alzheimer's disease is trouble with recent memory. It is not the "pathognomonic" that is equivalent with the diagnostic, but is a warning sign that a person can develop a memory illness in the coming years and therefore, together with their family, the individual should be vigilant in detecting the illness early and in rapid initiation of the specific treatment. On the other hand, not everyone with emerging memory problems will develop dementia; after all, forgetting is a part of everyday life and is sometimes a defense mechanism against negative events in life.

First possible "visible" signs to the patient or the family could be a state of sadness or a behavioral disorder (rarely in Alzheimer's disease but more frequently in dementia with Lewy bodies) or even a personality disorder (in frontotemporal dementia).

Some recent studies show the possibility of initial signs of impaired visual-praxis, meaning adaptation to different activities in spatial coordination, more simply said, errors in perceiving distances, for example such as, the emerging difficulties in parking one's car or space orientation with a map.

In the practical plan of this illness initiation, one can include repetition of the same questions, memory lapses (forgetting words while speaking fluently) or some bizarre actions like putting a shoe or the keys in the refrigerator.

Another rarer possibility, can be an episode of "transient global amnesia" (sometimes lasting for hours), whereby the patient is conscious and can conduct most diverse activities (including driving!), then not remembering anything from that period. Prior to this type of amnesia, a momentary forgetfulness can occur (the patient's empty stares, popularly "senior moments"), or repeated memory lapses becoming increasingly frequent.

Another possible situation, this time not encountered in the field of memory impairment, is the appearance at the onset of symptomatology, sometimes even before, of the olfaction distress (loss of the sense of smell) or, more rarely, of the taste for a large number of foods.

Any of these signs (cognitive, visual-spatial, smell) should be a warning to rapidly direct the pacient to a memory disorder specialist!

50. If you start forgetting in your fifties, does it mean that one will develop Alzheimer's?

As I mentioned in the previous question, not any cognitive impairment will lead to dementia, but if after the age of 50 years (sometimes earlier) you start to forget "differently" than before, it is mandatory to regularly meet a specialist in memory disorder, so as to assess the risk of developing this illness.

Even with the diagnosis of mild cognitive impairment (see Question 34), this does not necesarrily lead to a memory illness. It is true that in the first 5-6 years from making the diagnosis, over half of the patients will be diagnosed with dementia.

That is why it is so necessary to diagnose the "Alzheimer's disease" as early as possible, to take immediate measures to slow it down, because, as we know, at this moment there is no cure or treatment of these illnesses.

51. What are the clinical manifestations of the mild form of Alzheimer dementia?

According to DSM IV criteria, the specific clinical manifestations of dementia are:

1. Memory degeneration (impaired ability to take in new information or to recall previously recorded information)

2. One or more of the following cognitive disturbances:

a) Aphasia (language disturbance - verbal communication in the absence of strokes affecting the brain motor area)

b) Apraxia (impaired ability to perform a motor activity despite of intact motor functions)

c) Agnosia (inability to recognize or identify objects despite of unaffected sensory functions)

d) Disruption of the executive function (the ability to carry out projects, to organize in time, to have an abstract thinking)

The clinical evolution in dementia, according to this definition, is characterized by gradual onset and a continuous cognitive decline. Hence, the evolution is slow and the transition from a clinical form to another (from mild into the medium or frommedium into the severe form) is difficult to be observed in the absence of performing specific differentiation psychological tests.

Retrogenesis is considered the main clinical feature of Alzheimer's illness: this is a process which reverses the order of neuropsychological cognitive accumulations which have occurred during the active life of the individual, up to their complete loss, eventually. forgetting certain foreign languages happens in reverse relative to learning, the maternal language being the last to be forgotten.

However, from the clinical observations in large groups of patients, certain characteristics have been observed, which are more commonly found in a mild rather than medium form, as well as between a medium and severe form of dementia. Thus, in the mild stage, recent memory and language are deficient in some more complex discussions. Occasionally, the patient has difficulty following some TV shows.

The patient may have difficulties in indicating their age and/or their occupation prior to retirement. Sometimes, he/she could be cranky when carrying out more elaborate intellectual activities and even abandon them. The patient may be sad, apathetic and can sometimes easily cry, as well as react disinhibited under emotionally stress.

They can perform daily activities, mostly independently.

52. What are the clinical manifestations of the medium form of Alzheimer dementia?

The patient in the medium form of dementia is temporally confused (knows the season, but does not know the day, month and/or year), also possibly spatially (can get lost, not knowing the way home from previously known places).

More or less occasionally, they cannot remember the names of family members or family composition (how many children, how many grandchildren).

In everyday speech, although the language is obviously depleted for those who know them, sometimes the patient can digress or use inadequate words. They may react in an uninhibited manner to moderate emotional stimuli, up to psychomotor agitation and even verbal and physical violence.

Although the patient is still active, the person requires constant surveillance and support for some daily activities.

53. What are the clinical manifestations of the severe form of Alzheimer dementia?

The severe form of Alzheimer's disease, although obvious for a specialist, due to the evolution of this insidious illness, may not worry in the same extent a member of the family who is taking care of and has gradually taken over the functions of the patient in order to provide some relief. Thus, sadly, often the patient is first brought to the doctor in this stage, especially when he is in a family of intellectuals in which the patient dissimulates and masks the cognitive impairment for a long period.

The patient is disoriented both temporally and spatially, even with respect to their own identity, also not recognizing close acquaintances. It is not often that we have seen in the context of the patient's interview some family members being surprised by the wrong answers to some simple questions in this area of interest!

Recent memory is completely lost, the power of concentration being so low that the patient cannot carry on a simple conversation. His language is very poor, the patients failing to name the objects that are displayed to them.

The nycthemeral rhythm (sleep-waking rhythm) gets reversed, which emphasizes behavioral disorders occurring at this stage, panic attacks, anxiety and violence, mostly during the evenings (the phenomenon of the sun-downing).

In this final stage, the patient is completely dependent upon their caregivers.

Thus, terminal illness patient becomes abulic (inability to act, inertia), with bed confinement, and secondary pathology (strokes, infections, bedsores), with deglutition disorders, mutism. In the end, from a neurogical standpoint, only the archaic reflections remain (sucction or grip reflex, also known as holding) which are characteristics of the newborn.

54. Can clinical manifestations vary depending on the time of day?

Patients with Alzheimer dementia may be more nervous at sundown (sundowning syndrome) and can develop psychomotor agitation leading up to verbal and even physical violence in the hours following behavioral disorders. The phenomenon is present in 1 in 5 patients with dementia in medium/severe and severe phases, disturbing the nycthemeral rhythm (sleep-wake alternation). Its cause is still unknown but it is assumed to be due to the accumulated fatigue during the day or of distressed "internal clock". In some cases, the identification of restless legs syndrome, UTI or urinary incontinence which disrupt the patient's sleep, through the treatment of these causes, the sundowning syndrome can be also solved.

The treatment of sleep and behaviour disorders should be made only with the recommendation of a specialist, otherwise there is a risk of worsening the problems.

On the other hand, there are many patients presenting a confusing state in the morning, when they wake up, considering that the phenomenon is the result of an increased degree of ischemia, particularly at the level of the posterior circulation of the brain to the transition from sleep into wakefulness. Thus, they may not recognize their surroundings momentarily, or their family members. As I mentioned before, the phenomenon is transient and disappears without the need of any intervention.

55. *Does sexual desire diminish or disappear in patients with dementia?*

This topic is avoided most of the time, including discussions with a patient's own doctor. It is a highly complex subject, even taboo in some cultures, when referring to the elderly and involves different connotations.

Given the different degree of neurological damage from one patient to another, it is difficult to draw general conclusions.

However, it is clear that for some patients, the sexual desire persists while it might disappear for others. Another situation is that of the patients that show a sexual disinhibition caused by the illness, which may result in many unusual situations, some even with a forensic connotation.

In the case of some stable couples, the appearance of Alzheimer dementia in one of the partners, even with a slow, gradual, evolution, makes intimate activity possible in, or near, the same conditions as before. Usually, in such couples the sexual activity interruption occurs when the partner-caregiver finds an impairment of judgement in the patient – lack of the partner's judgement but also the lack of pleasure.

A delicate situation is that of institutionalized patients who are undergoing sexual abuse, sometimes advantage being taken of their sexual disinhibition. Here, the role of institution leadership on permanent supervision of patients as well as of the staff, is important.

It is usually the role of the psychologist to carry out an investigation in this area, in order to identify possible causes of misunderstandings and sometimes of conflicts within the couple. Often, I had aged couples in which both partners were affected by the illness to a greater or lesser extent, case in which the family must be informed about these situations which require measures, sometimes even their separate care.

56. Currently, are there reversible or curable types of dementia?

Dementia, despite the popular idea of its incurability (i.e. illness without a curative treatment), may be reversible when caused by some medications, alcohol, malnutrition, hormonal imbalances and vitamin deficiencies, depression, as well as by some other causes (sensorial deprivation –reduction or lack of hearing or sight, sleep apnea). In this context, it is important to thoroughly evaluate the patient's symptoms to detect potentially treatable conditions.

The frequency of reversible dementias is evaluated by different authors to be between 1-20% (high variability). The most important neurological treatment coordinated by the reputed professor of neurology Raymond Adams, states that 10% of patients directed to neurology centers have reversible metabolic disorders or psychiatric illnesses. Early recognition of reversible dementia can determine its healing, with all positive implications at the individual and community level. Until recently there has been a limited interest in the differential diagnosis expanded beyond exclusion of "traditionally" reversible dementias.

"Globalization" of the dementias, in which all dementias are simplistically classified as "Alzheimer", brings an incorrect diagnostic for a while and some other times, unfortunately, the diagnostic of reversible dementia to be determined too late, when it can no longer influence the illness, or at the histopathological examination of the brain after death.

Any suspected dementia syndrome must entail a standardized psychometric assessment and asset of tests in order to exclude:

a) "traditionally" reversible dementias (severe depression usually with a chronic background, of melancholy type), brain tumors - primary or secondary (metastatic), hypothyroidism, deficit of vitamin B12 and/or folic acid.

b) certain types of rarer reversible dementia, due to certain pathological conditions: vitamin B1 deficit, HIV-AIDS that causes AIDS-dementia complex, syphilis, Creutzfeld-Jakobs illness dementia, intoxication with certain substances – aluminum, hypoxia accentuated in severe cardiac and respiratory illnesses, severe dehydration, hepatic encephalopathy, normal pressure hydrocephalus, cerebral hematoma- usually subdural, posttraumatic severe sensorial deficits – the so-called sensorial deprivation through impaired sight and hearing.

All these pathological conditions, once diagnosed and treated, can cause partial or total reversal of the cognitive symptoms.

The differential diagnostic, i.e. selecting the correct diagnostic, includes the following elements:

A) Evaluation of duration, frequency and rate of progression of symptoms and the patient's detailed history (including administered medication) but also family history - i.e. if the patient has a first degree relative who suffered from Alzheimer's disease

B) Assessment of the presence of a history of depression, substance abuse (voluntarily or non-voluntarily, chronic or acute) or heart, pulmonary, hormonal, kidney and/or liver illnesses.

C) The dosage of vitamin B1, hemoglobin, vitamin B12, folic acid and homocysteine in blood, thyroid hormones and thyroid regulators (T3, T4, TSH), of serotonin levels (for depression), certain blood serial glycemia (possibility of a latent, unknown or neglected diabetes).

D) The presence of bacteria/viruses (which will be detailed below) or greater quantity of metals in blood.

E) Imaging tests (brain, heart, lung, thyroid, liver, kidney) for

the diagnosis of comorbidities (concurrent illnesses) that can influence or even cause dementia.
F) Clinical examination (including detailed neurology) performed on apparatus and systems, in which the doctor's experience and flair are very important in a maybe too technogical world.

G) Standardized psychometric evaluation, dynamically performed (tests at given intervals) by a psychologist or experienced psychogeriatrician
H) Ophthalmologic examination for evidence and resolution of possible ocular causes known for worsening the cognitive impairment (cataracts, glaucoma), as well as an ENT examination with the same purpose. A simple algorithm, which can be followed during the investigation of the reversible causes, is based on etiology (cause of the illness):

- The elimination of the causes of malignancy (i.e. the possibility of a brain tumor).

- The elimination of the infectious causes (bacterial, viral and sometimes fungal infections).

- The elimination of the autoimmune causes (autoimmune illnesses gain an increasingly higher importance, with the development of immunology).

- The elimination of the metabolic and toxic causes (including vitamin deficits).

- The elimination of the vascular causes (which in principle cannot be excluded given the changes in the small vessels of the brain and neurodegenerative illnesses, such as Alzheimer dementia and vascular dementia).

There are several reversible causes of dementia that can be grouped into a mnemonic formula in the **DEMENTIA** term, for easier memorization:

Drugs - basically, any medication with anticholinergic action may cause cognitive impairment.

Emotional – depression.

Metabolic – the most common cause of hypothyroidism.

Eyes and ears declining – sensorial visual and/or audible deprivation.

Normal pressure hydrocephalus.

Tumor or other space – occupying brain lesion.

Infection (syphilis, AIDS).

Anemia – vitamin B12 and/or folic acid deficit.

To continue, I will give details about some reversible pathological conditions that are met more frequently in the medical practice.

Severe endocrine disorders and the deficit of certain vitamins can "stimulate" a dementia and necessitates their investigation, especially in the precocious dementias with a rapid evolution.

Hypothyroidism – A recent study showed a statistically valid correlation between a TSH greater than 2.1 and the risk of developing a dementia (the correlation is with Alzheimer's dementia in the study). The diagnosis can be made fast through a trivial dosing of certain markers of the thyroid function from the blood (T3, T4 – the thyroid hormones and TSH – pituitary hormone that regulates T3 and T4).

Normal serum values: TSH – 0.27 – 4.20 µUI/mL

T3 – 0.83 – 2 NG/Ml

T4 – 5.13 – 14.1 µg/dL

The deficit of vitamin B12 (cobalamin)

- Caused by alcoholism, Crohn disease, celiac disease.
- Characterized by apathy, irritability, sluggishness and confusion, alteration of perspicacity and abstract thinking, atrophy of the optic nerve and peripheral neuropathy and in the end dementia.
- False decreases: folate deficiency – the values normalize folowing a folate treatment; it has to be differentiated from the combinaed deficit of both vitamins.

Normal serum values Vitamin B12 – 191-663 pmol/L.

- **The deficit of vitamin B1 (thiamine)** – The precocious signs of thiamine deficit include anorexia, weight loss, muscular hypotonia, apathy, confusion and irritability. The late manifestations of the deficit are congestive cardiac insufficiency ("wet Beri-Beri"), polyneuropathy with diminished reflexes, paresthesia, muscular atrophy ("dry Beri-Beri") and Wernicke-Korsakoff syndrome, characterized by dementia, ataxia and ophthalmoplegia.

Normal serum values of vitamin B1 – 40 – 49 μg/L.

Normal pressure hydrocephalus (NPH) has a prevalence of 21.9 cases for 100 000 residents, being a form of reversible dementia characterized by a clinical triad:

- cognitive deficit (of frontal and subcortical type),

- walking disorders (shamble walk with an enlarged support base),

- urinary incontinence.

Imaging evaluation (CT or MRI) emphasizes a ventriculomegaly (a dilatation of certain cerebral structures named ventricles). The classification of normal pressure hydrocephalus is made in two ways:

- Idiopathic, present in the elderly (chronic NPH) with an insidious debut or even silent.

- Symptomatic (secondary), with acute or chronic debut.

    - subarachnoid hemorrhage (aneurism),

    - post-infectious,

    - post-traumatic.

NPH treatment is surgical through insertion of ventricular shunt, most of the time achieving a communication between the brain and the abdominal cavity, for the decrease of the hydrocephalus. The diagnostic tests cannot predict the postoperative results, but most of the time the results are very good (the disappearance of dementia!). *On the other hand, numerous potentially reversible conditions can be associated with a cognitive deficit without being included in the criteria for specific dementia.*

The variability is very great in appreciating the frequency of reversible dementias between different authors (between 1-20%) and it emphasizes the necessity of having a well-structured guide of evaluation of dementias that can also take into consideration the differential diagnosis with these rarer, yet potentially treatable forms of dementia.

57. How early should the treatment of this illness begin?

Of course, as with any illness, the treatment should be started even before the first symptoms for the so-called "patients at risk", this type of treatment representing the primary prevention. Any person who has a close relative (a parent, grandparent, brother or sister) who has had or has dementia must reflect on how to prevent or delay its appearance as much as possible.

Also, those people suffering from certain illnesses at least susceptible to different types of dementia and especially vascular dementia (hypertension, diabetes, dyslipidemic illness, especially hypercholesterolemia – the "bad cholesterol" i.e. LDL - cholesterol is increased either with a concurrent or decrease in the "good cholesterol" HDL or not, i.e. obesity, smoking - chronic smoking) are now considered "patients at risk". All these illnesses cause damage to the blood vessels especially the arterioles (smallest arteries) including at the brain level, which over time will lead to the death of neurons by blocking blood flow to neurons, and consequently to mild cognitive impairment and thereafter dementia.

Considering that at this moment there is no treatment (to cure the disease), the question arises whether this effort of primary prevention of the illness is useful. Although there are a number of research projects in this regard, they take time to be be converted into "value judgments". However, theoretically, *any action that would result in reducing risk factors could cause the delay of the illness, with benefits at both the individual level (for the same average lifespan, a later occurrence of dementia would result in a shorter period of illness) but also for the community (reducing overall costs with the illness).* In other words, as Dr. Craft at Washington University was stating, delaying the onset of illness five years later would half the new cases of the illness, given that most occur after the age of 80.

Thus, a number of different classes of antihypertensive agents (diuretics, enzyme converting inhibitors of angiotensin, calcium blockers, etc.) may be used to bring systolic and diastolic blood pressure within normal parameters (140 mmHg systolic, 90 mmHg diastolic), as recommended by the geriatrician, cardiologist, internist or family doctor.

In order to keep the blood glucose levels as close to normal as possible (105-115 mg/dl, according to the investigating laboratory reference values), especially for a patient already diagnosed with diabetes, an appropriate diet is recommended (reducing the amount of carbohydrates and expecially sweets), physical exercise and diabetes treatment (oral agents and/or insulin) when needed and recommended by a doctor specializing in nutritional and diabetes.

Also, in case of hypercholesterolemia (resulting from an inadequate intake of fat and/or familial illness) – for values of total cholesterol over 200 mg/dl and LDL – cholesterol greater than 100 mg/dl, a hypolipidic diet is recommended (especially without animal fats, i.e. no processed meat, sausages, pork, non-skimmed milk) – and possibly, the administration of lipid-lowering medication (statins).

58. Who are the doctors who can help?

In every country, there should be a specific approach to Alzheimer's pathology. Unfortunately, the huge costs of a systematic action in the field still make this a desire rather than a reality...

For example, in Europe there are some more developed countries with a "National Alzheimer Program", which standardizes both specific approach and the patients' and caregivers' support. In less developed countries (such as in Eastern Europe) the approach is generally chaotic and differs greatly from country to country.

However, when viewed as a whole, the approach should involve all specialists (neurologists, psychiatrists, geriatricians), as well as general practitioners who should be its cornerstone. Why am I saying this? Because if every GP could identify the risk factors, as they were presented in the previous question, or the early appearance of a cognitive impairment (any disorder of memory may be a start sign), the general practicioner should immediately refer the patient to a specialist for investigation. Of course, in those countries where this does not happen, the family or the individual himself who suspects a cognitive impairment must look for a specialist to act as quickly as possible.

Equally important is the educational role of these popular books in general cognitive pathology and dementia Alzheimer's and other types of dementia in particular. It is not enough to develop a complex scientific approach to Alzheimer's pathology if we don't care about its implementation within the general population, those with a lower level of education.

59. What tests must be done first? What about later?

The first tests which should be conducted in case of cognitive impairment being suspected are those performed by a clinical psychologist or a doctor who specializes in diagnosing the illness. These can lead us to a "mild cognitive impairment under observation" diagnosis or even dementia, according to standardized values obtained from this evaluation.

Intellectual performance – cognitive tests most frequently used:

• **Mini Mental State Examination** is evaluated according to the educational level (EL), with different values for low *EL and high **EL (where *EL corresponds to primary education and **EL to secondary education or higher). It is the most important and most commonly used memory test, being fast enough and investigating main areas of cognition (including as they are diagnosed within the new DSM V assessment of dementia), respectively attention and concentration, short-term memory language, executive functions and praxia.

• The clock test - the patient draws the face of a clock with all the hours and then indicates the precise time. The maximum score is 10 points.

• Verbal Fluency - the patient lists from memory in one minute as many words semantically belonging to a group as possible.

• The Rey Scheme – the patient copies and after a few minutes draws a complex drawing from memory.

• The Grober-Buscke Test - the patient learns a list of 18 words and then calls them out twice successively from memory.

The scores on these assessments take into account the prior educational level and cognitition of the patient. **An evaluation through these tests is presented in Appendix 12.**

In practice, we also use the "test of 10 words", which is a rapid test that involves viewing 10 cards, each containing one word (a fairly familiar object) which the patient should reproduce. This process is repeated 3 times and the results from three averaged exercises. A score at least equal to 7 is considered acceptable.

Its worth mentioning other cognitive tests, most notably ADAS-COG, a very useful test, but whose duration is approximately one hour, thus involving a longer time dedicated to each patient.

There are other tests used quite frequently in diagnosing memory illnesses and associated symptoms, such as NPI - Neuro - Psychiatric Inventory (diagnosing disorders of psychiatric type) GDS - Geriatric depression scale (differential diagnosis of depression with cognitive elements).

Also, it is important for the evaluation to be carried out when the patient is at rest (usually in the morning), in a quiet enviroment and ensuring discretion and professional confidentiality.

In the last 10-15 years, the cognitive as well as the functional assessment could be achieved using standardized scales, for instance: the cognitive impairment scale rate, clinic dementia scale, global deterioration scale.

Cognitive Impairment Rating Scale (CIRS)

This scale helps determining the rate of cognitive impairment severity in five cognitive domains with five levels of severity.

The score is based on the history as described by the patient, caregivers or observations during the subject interview. In case of discrepancy between different sources, the highest level of severity between the three sources is being used.

The five areas used are: memory, language, executive functions, visual praxia, attention and concentration as the last field.

The five levels of severity are: normal, very easy, easy, medium and severe.

In the field of memory, the five levels of severity are:

- **Level 1** – Immediate and recent memory unaffected
- **Level 2** – Very easy: occasional misplacing items and retrieving them later, trouble remembering a phone number, forgetting some details about a recent event or forgetting a recent event but recalling it on different occasions
- **Level 3** – Easy: sometimes misplacing items, repetition of stories or questions, frequently forgetting some details of recent events or important meetings, the person has no

shopping list and forgets to buy certain items, sometimes forget their medication, have trouble learning how to use new devices (home appliances, computer, etc)

- **Level 4** – Medium: Occasionally disoriented in time or space, sometimes lost in a common environment, often forgetting recent events, often repeating stories or questions, often forgetting to take medication, sometimes forgetting how to perform household chores
- **Level 5** – Severe: Disoriented in time and space, often not being able to handle familiar situations, most often forgetting recent events or stories, often repeated questions, requiring permanent assistance for daily activity

Clinical Dementia Rating Scale - CDR

This scale examines six areas with five levels of severity.

The analyzed areas are: memory, orientation, problem solving, social activities, household chores and hobbies, personal care.

The 5 levels of severity are: normal (0 pts.), very easy (0.5 pts.), easy (1 pt.), medium (2pts.), severe (3 pts.).

Global Deterioration Scale (GDS)

This scale is conducted by an experienced investigator as a function of data collected during the structured, standardized assessment.

The scale has seven levels: normal, very easy, easy, moderate, moderate - severe, severe, very severe.

The simple way to evaluate a patient with dementia is achieved by using the Activity of Daily Living (ADL) and more complexely by Instrumental Activity of Daily Living (IADL-see Appendix 7).

Activity daily living (ADL) - the daily activity of the subject.

Six items are taken into consideration: personal hygiene, dressing, going to the toilet, locomotion, continence, meals.

For each item: one, two or three points are assigned for autonomy, the need for aid and partly that total dependence on another person respectively.

For light cognitive impairment, the score of 6 points should be achieved by subjects who present no disabilities prior to the occurrence of cognitive impairment.

IADL (Instrumental Activity of Daily Living) – regular complex activities of the subject.

Eight items are taken into account: the ability to use one's phone, go shopping, prepare food, household maintenance, washing clothes, using transportation, responsibility towards the ongoing treatment, ability to use money. Each item is scored 0 or 1 point based on different criteria for each item.

In the mild cognitive impairment, the asymptomatic preclinical stage of patients without cognitive impairment should score 8 points if all items can be used (e.g. items as cooking, washing clothes are not always applied for men).

Generally, each "memory center" has its own approach to assessing cognition of their patients, given the time necessary for a consultation center and the experience gained by that center in these evaluation types.

With the evolution of illness, the assessment area narrows down, and the examiner's experience becomes crucial in establishing a diagnosis closer to that resulting after the autopsy examination, establishing a prognosis of illness (survival time) and especially an appropriate treatment.

60. Are the imagistic tests mandatory from the beginning?

The imaging tests are not necessary for the initial assessment, considering that even those less expensive, such as brain tomography, are not very relevant (there is dementia without cortical atrophy but also cortical atrophy presents in people who do not suffer from dementia) and the most complex (positron emission tomography, functional imaging) are too expensive to be routinely performed.

Computed tomography of the brain determines the encephal aspect and the subcortical structures, both at the gray and white matter level. It can detect brain atrophy (decrease of the volumetric brain and possibly of the cerebellum), hydrocephalus, stroke and lacunar stroke. Nuclear magnetic resonance examination has more fidelity, as it highlights damages much smaller than tomography can achieve, but is more expensive than the former. Likewise, by using magnetic resonance, studies of brain volumetry can be achieved and also functional imagery for the focused stimulation of different brain areas.

There is also the possibility of an MR angiography with a detailed visualization of blood circulation at the Willis polygon level (a brain communication structure of the anterior and posterior circulation of the brain) and also of the circulatory tree which irrigates the brain structures (carotids and anterior, medium and posterior cerebral arteries).

Some studies have established terms of predictive and diagnostic accuracy for performance imaging (PET, SPECT). PET and SPECT examinations in the parietal-temporal cortex highlight metabolic disorders.

Predictivity has showed decreased perfusion or metabolism of glucose in:

- The parietal and temporal lobes.
- The posterior cingulate gyrus.
- The frontal lobe.

Diagnostic accuracy in these studies was higher for both PET and SPECT as compared to CT and MRI.

The recommendation for a specific imaging investigation rests with the specialist doctor depending on the patient's cognitive impairment. Unfortunately, not everywhere is the functional imaging part of the health insurance programs and thus requires direct payment. Also, at some time interval the imagistic evaluation is repeated in order to quantify structural but also functional brain changes with the disease evolution, or may be repeated when there is worsening of the illness or brain related vascular pathology ("straight" stroke – i.e. noticeable signs and symptoms).

61. Should environmental changes for patients with dementia be avoided?

Changing environment (including hospitalization in a Center, accountancy) can sometimes accelerate the evolution of this illness (ischemic strokes occur - acute myocardial infarction, acute stroke - impaired psychomotor agitation - behavioral, intercurrent infections amid a weakened immune system, sometimes with saprofiti germs, that is). After a period of approx. 2-3 weeks, usually the patient adjusts to the new environment. Unfortunately, there are also cases in which evolution is sometimes negative, leading up to death.

Only the specialist may specify when and how it should be actioned in the case of a patient with dementia. In the case of medium/severe or severe dementia patients, I recommend a short-term hospitalization (3-5 days) for a complex evaluation of the cognitive and behavioral status, and after psychological counseling (both with the patient and family) to establish the risk degree of a long-term or even permanent institutionalization in a specialized centre.

Institutionalization of patients in advanced stages of the illness should be performed after the patient's relatives are being explained, on one hand the perspective for the patient to remain with the family (when possible) and, on the other hand, of patient's integration in a suitable environment coordinated by professionals in the field, but also the risks related to these decisions.

62. Can a patient have dementia and depression at the same time?

It has to be known that any patient may have comorbidities (i.e. several illnesses at the same time), so that even in theory, the association between depression and dementia is possible.

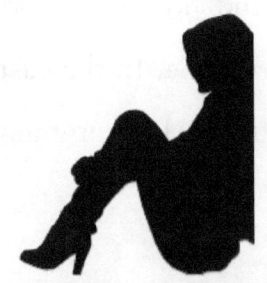

In medical practice the combination of the two entities is fairly common. Evaluating their chronology is important because of the known possibility of a so-called "dementia with depressive features" and also a so-called "depression with cognitive element". In fact, the coexistence of two concurrent implies their concurrent treatment. On the other hand, there are antidepressant – tianeptine – drugs with positive effects on cognition as "neuroplasticity" (the brain's ability to reorganize itself in order to form new neuronal connections).

Throughout my professional activity I have seen several cases diagnosed with dementia (sometimes in a severe form!) usually accompanied by apathy, who responded favorably to a sustained antidepressant treatment, (in one case over a few years). Certainly, there are plenty of depressions (either severe or with a long evolution) which are diagnosed as dementia.

63. May depression precede dementia?

There is a depression that precedes dementia, sometimes as a preamble or as the first sign of dementia but there is the possibility of a depression pre-existing dementia, hence with no causal relationship with it. Often the anamnesis review of a patient with dementia has revealed that they displayed sometimes even decades before, a depressive episode or recurrent depression which had gone untreated, or insufficiently treated or whose treatment was discontinued on their own specific will.

There are patients who have maintained a lifetime depression, melancholy, and whom at old age develop a degenerative type dementia (Alzheimer's). They show "somatization" disorders meaning symptoms that have no organic cause (burning sensation on the tip of your tongue, tingling throughout the body, etc.), long before the appearance of memory disorders. Sometimes such patients are considered hypochondriacs (i.e. "The Imaginary Invalid"), but time has proven that these events were part of the onset of the illness.

64. What are the most common behavioral disorders in dementia?

Along with intellectual functions and functional abilities, behavior disorders are part of the clinical triad of dementias. In medical practice, most often, the latter are "warning shots" which convince even the most skeptical family members about the diagnosis, so as to bring the patient to the doctor. Unfortunately, at least in Alzheimer dementia, behavioral disturbances occur late when restoring a functional balance becomes unlikely.

The following symptoms will be treated:
- psychomotor agitation
- The verbal and/or physical aggression
- Delusional, persecution or prejudicial ideas

A good medical practice in the field means:
- Defining the symptoms
- Carefully choosing the specific medication, respecting the adverse event profile
- The loading dose must be reduced and daily dosage be gradually increased
- Tracking the response and side effects, both on short and long term
- The administration of medication to be initiated closest to the onset of symptoms
- Sometimes the evening dose should be administered separately from the rest of medication prior to the evening meal and to the potential sun-downing type phenomena that occur after 5 o'clock p.m.

To treat or not to treat?
- This is a very important question (Primum non nocere - First, do not harm)

- Does the patient shows symptoms? Is the caregiver's information correct?
- It can be difficult to tell the difference between "I think he/she sees things" and "sees things"
- Does the symptom cause a real inconvenience - and for whom? Is the patient affected by this symptom, or the caregivers?
- Is another cause possible? (Delirium for example)?
- Is a behavioral management possible?

Psychosis has a high prevalence in Alzheimer dementia considering the medium and severe stages (illusions in about 30% of cases, hallucinations in 1 of 5 cases).

Dementia with Lewy bodies is typically associated with visual hallucinations which are present in an increasing number of cases.

Psychosis is associated with aggression and psychomotor agitation.

Medication used to treat behavioral disorders is mainly of antipsychotic type.

During the course of the antipsychotic treatment evolution, typical neuroleptics have been used initially and subsequently in order to reduce atypical side effects (18/100 patients with dementia receive neuroleptic therapy).

The characteristics of the first-generation antipsychotics therapy (typical neuroleptics):

• Initially, haloperidol has been used as antipsychotic therapy in behavioral disturbances of dementia

• Low Potential antipsychotic (thioridazine, Chlorpromazine) having anticholinergic, sedative and hypotensive properties

• Potential increased of walking troubles (haloperidol) causes more frequently extrapyramidal side effects

Characteristics of the second-generation antipsychotic therapy (atypical neuroleptics):

• Antipsychotic effects much improved over the previous generation

• Determine greatly reduced side effects relative to typical neuroleptics in the following areas:

- Cognitive impairment

- Hypotension

- Extrapyramidal side effects.

If the treatment is unavoidable, then the atypical antipsychotics are less harmful but the loading dose should be minimal, gradually increasing, then reducing it once the effect is achieved down to the minimum efficient limit!

I have not detailed here the antipsychotic medication for a single purpose: that of awareness that this type of medication can only be administered by a psychiatrist or psychogeriatrician, considering the serious side effects which can occur when using them. The emergence of such symptomatology is an urgent and immediate need to direct the patient to a medical specialist!

65. When can behavioral disorders occur in the illness?

Behavioral and personality disorders can sometimes occur before cognitive symptoms (impaired memory, thinking, judgment) being confused with other psychiatric illnesses and determining erroneous treatment options.

In broad strokes, behavioral disorders can occur from subcortical dementia onset amid a personality disorder, constantly accompanied by bradypsychia.

In cortical dementias, the cognitive function disorders are sometimes preceded by emotional control disorders, personality changes, or psychiatric symptoms (apathy, depression, psychotic disorders) and behavioral disorders.

Most often however, behavioral disorders occur late in medium/severe and severe form of the illness.

66. Can the caregivers' behavior influence the illness?

The stress, experienced because of care for patients with dementia, can lead to changes in behavior of family members (caregivers), who, through the interaction with the patient (verbal and sometimes even physical violence), may cause degradation of the patient's physical condition. Diametrically opposed to this the evolution of the disease can be clearly influenced by carefully attending to the patient's needs, especially in terms of improving the patient's quality of life.

From my professional experience, I recall two cases in which the relationship between caregiver (referring to family members) and patient had become conflictual leading up to physical violence. In one particular case, the daughter (a person with high educational level) admitted that she hit her mother in a crisis situation, and the other phenomenon was so striking that the patient, although in an advanced stage of illness, stated the fear of being molested as an echolalia (repeating a sentence or a phrase) related to the trauma she has been repeatedly subject to.

Of course, **the deterioration of the relationship between caregiver and patient is caused by increased physical disability, but especially given the conditions of the onset of behavioral troubles for the patient, which often are very hard to counteract.**

Assessment of caregivers for patients with dementia can be done through various tests, one of which best known is the Zarit Burden Interview (main caregiver burden assessment).

67. *How can we help caregivers cope with the situation?*

It is important to conduct educational programs for caregivers to understand the natural evolution of the illness but also be mentally prepared for its final stages, when the stress level is high.

Unfortunately, not all countries possess a national program in place for patients with Alzheimer dementia, as to provide both financial and moral support to their families. Most often, the role of this national program is assumed by various non-governmental organizations which can not, normally achieve a coherent coordination of actions for patients and their caregivers.

Thus, an important role is incumbent on specialists, especially psychologists and psychiatrists but also psychogeriatricians involved in the field. Knowing the precise evolution of the illness helps the family overcome more easily both psychological and physical changes, so unexpected for a family member who until recently was a healthy active person.

Creating support groups, made up of professionals but also patients' families, with regular (weekly or bi-weekly) meetings can very useful in support of this goal.

68. Can impaired sleep influence the illness?

The problem of sleep disorders is an important issue between the manifestations of dementia in general and Alzheimer dementia in particular. The most important consequence of these nyctothemeral rhythm changes (alternating normal sleep-wake cycle) is the fall, with all the complications that derive from it. The main complication encountered (especially in women, due to the increased incidence of osteoporosis, as compared to men) is the femur fracture (especially at the femoral neck), which implies surgery as a therapeutic approach, with a low frequency of healing. In addition, general anesthesia may cause a worsening of cognitive impairment, often causing in these patients the impossibility of learning how to walk again. Thus, some of them remain bedridden, secondary mortality in the first year being 1 in 3 people who have experienced this situation (compared to 1 in 5 non-demented individuals who had an intervention of this kind).

Consequently, families of dementia patients should be advised how to prevent fracture risk by optimizing the environment and lives of people with dementia (larger spaces, furniture reduced to a minimum). Another major problem occurring in parallel, secondary to sleep disorders, are behavioral disorders, including the sundowning phenomenon (see Question 53). They lead to the administration by a specialist of antipsychotics and/or hypnotics, which increases the risk of falls and secondarily, achain of events presented previously leading up to premature death of the patient with dementia.

> Thus, a very judicious administration of these drugs is extremely important, by utilizing combinations thereof and minimal active doses, of course only as prescribed by the specialist!

69. What are the problems which the patient with dementia can cause?

The family often minimizes or even hides the behavioral disorders of patients with dementia (see Question 66). More dangerous is the situation whereby the caregivers do not recognize these disorders and therefore do not take steps to treat them. In all these cases, as in other illnesses with behavioral disorders, critical situations can emerge ranging up from suicide to murder.

In this context, the role of the specialist in explaining to the family the risk posed to both patients and surrounding individuals (family, if home care or medical personnel for the hospitalized patient) is very important, unless a specific treatment (usually an antipsychotic) is administered, adequate security measures (including constraint) are being taken. Although constraint is stipulated both in international law and the laws of most countries, constituting a safety measure necessary for some patients with psychomotor agitation or even violent, it requires a prior process of family counseling. The family will be explained the belt types being used, the location, the duration of their use (only during the period in which the patient can inflict self harm or affect the integrity of the persons in the immediate environment, but also to prevent the risk of falls). The period these measures are taken shall be recorded on the patient observation sheet, as well as the reasons for these steps.

On the other hand, a patient with dementia in either medium or severe stage, but who can move about, does require constant surveillance to avoid domestic or traffic accidents.

70. Can we delay its progression?

It is a question for which there is not yet an affirmative, proven answer! Researchers have launched a series of studies which are still ongoing, focused on this assessment, even considering the possibility of avoiding the illness through prevention programs, especially for people with a family history (see also Question 23).

The American Alzheimer Association is funding studies exploring the influence of various factors such as exercise, cognitive stimulation "mental fitness", diet, environmental factors, and vascular risk factors (see Questions 25-27 and 31). Some studies show that a particular factor may have some effect on an individual, but what is important is that the effect be applicable to the entire population.

The studies evaluating prevention and management of risk factors need to be performed on large samples of a healthy population over a long period of time (decades), which is both difficult and expensive. In the United States there are non-governmental organizations recruiting healthy volunteers to participate in such clinical trials.

71. *When should we consult a doctor for the first time?*

A first assessment of the cognitive (intellectual) functions by a specialist or psychologist - given recent evidence of Alzheimer's disease showing up at maturity already - should be performed at the age of 35-40. Thus, once the suspicion of possible evolution of a neurocognitive disorder (according to DSM V) is revealed, measures can be taken for preventing or slowing the progression of Alzheimer's disease (previous question).

Conducted tests will evaluate the retrograde memory, the temporal and spatial orientation, attention, concentration and verbal fluency, the visual praxis and the abstract thinking (see Question 59).

The general practitioner has an important role in illness detection, who should conduct a brief assessment when a patient complains of general impairment of cognition and memory in particular. Unfortunately, this rarely happens in the absence of a nationwide coherent program of early detection.

> We resume this topic because early diagnosis is the most important for the future of finding solutions to slow or even cure neurodegenerative dementing illnesses.

72. *What should the doctor look for on the first appointment?*

Be it with the general practitioner or the specialist (neurologist, psychiatrist, psychogeriatrician), the first consultation, conducted mostly at the request of the patient, must assess the patient's cognition as a whole, but not before performing a meticulous anamnesis, which takes into account the family illness history (parents, siblings), but also pathological personal antecedents (head injury sustained even in childhood, infectious states – infectious meningitis, syphilis, HIV – hypothyroidism, Cushing's disease, heart and serious respiratory illnesses) - see Questions 32, 33, 56).

Also to be assessed are the presence of illnesses considered risk factors such as hypertension, diabetes, hypercholesterolemia, obesity (see Questions 25, 26, 27, 31).

The patient will be asked about psycho-social factors in their life, about their addictions (smoking, alcohol), as well as signs and symptoms they display (evaluated by monitoring the devices and systems thereof, otherwise the patient may skip the ones they deem irrelevant or simply the ones they forget!).

The clinical consultation should be thorough, including a neurological exam at both the central but also the peripheral nervous system.

The doctor will evaluate abstract thinking and memory constantly during the interview by asking for details and locations of temporal and spatial events described by the patient, discreetly, without the patient realizing it. This will help the patient to take a relaxed approach and make a connection with the doctor, which can be consolidated long-term.

If after that first consultation, as a result of professional experience, the doctor considers that the person has no cognitive impairment and no predisposition to a mental disease, he will recommend them only general prevention measures (reduction of vascular risk factors) and a revaluation for next year.

If the person shows symptoms of mild cognitive impairment (see Question 34), the doctor will direct the patient to a specific neuropsychological evaluation (see question 59) and paraclinical laboratory investigations necessary for a more precise positive diagnosis (see Question 60).

Medical reassessments for patients with cognitive impairment in/or outside the dementias will be made in accordance with a well-established program by the attending physician (see Question 73).

73. At what interval should the patient be re-evaluated?

The first very important aspect is that the patient must strictly present themselves for revaluation at the interval specified by the physician. There is a tendency to delay the revaluation if the patient has a favorable evolution, with possible negative effects of the illness.

The second aspect is that each doctor sets the time, based on: personal experience, the patient's condition at the time of consultation, stage of illness and the presence of more serious symptoms, such as behavioral disorders (hallucinations, delusions).

From personal experience, I recommend for a mild cognitive impairment for the revaluation to be done annually and at dementia onset, reassessments at 6 months and then every 3 months or as needed (agitation, sleep disorders, etc.) in advanced stages of the illness.

Of course, in the terminal stages of dementia, the evaluation will be performed regularly, ideally daily in an institutionalized environment.

74. Are there any signs which can confirm the diagnosis of Alzheimer dementia?

Firstly, from a nosological standpoint (nosology – the branch of medicine that studies illnesses in general), what we are looking for in a diagnosis of dementia are not signs but symptoms that correlate with it. Thus, the right question is "Are there symptoms which confirm the diagnostics of dementia?" The answer is yes and no! Because although there are some symptoms which correlate in a larger proportion with Alzheimer dementia diagnostics sustained until the death of the patient, at the necropsy the microscopic examination of the brain, other changes specific to other types of dementia can be also highlighted (vascular, frontotemporal, Lewy body).

However, given the relatively large correlation, we can state that in the presence of cognitive impairment (memory disorders, language and praxia) which emerges insidioulsy and shows a gradual evolution, severe enough to affect the patient on a daily basis, but in the absence of neurological syndromes (pyramidal, extrapyramidal, cerebellar), the diagnostics is Alzheimer dementia.

75. *Should the patient with dementia be treated from the beginning?*

The answer is yes and, at risking of repeating myself, early diagnosis and quickly initiated specific treatment are key to the illness evolution. Thus, *extending the period in which the patient is active, it is useful on both the individual and community level by shortening the final period when the patient is bedridden, and involves greatly reduced costs both morally and pecuniary.*

Once diagnosis of dementia is made, it requires specific treatment initiation, which unfortunately does not cure the illness (see Question 79).

76. *Are there any drugs that cure this illness?*

The answer is unfortunately NO if we think of a curative treatment, that is a treatment which can heal the illness. Dozens of researches have been conducted in the past 20 years worldwide but, unfortunately, none has resulted in a miracle treatment that can reverse the illness in the case of neurodegenerative dementias.

Current therapeutic possibilities, in neurodegenerative dementias, are classified by their action mode into:

• symptomatic – clinical improvement without modifying the illness progression (see Question 79);

• possibly active – specific illness pathophysiological events (see Questions 79, 80, 81);

• preventive – initiation before the appearance of clinical signs of the illness (see Question 57).

As for the *reversible dementias* (see Question 56), their early recognition can determine healing (by rapidly treating its cause), with all the positive implications at the individual and community levels.

77. Should certain medications be avoided in the treatment of dementia?

As we know, all drugs have some positive effects and many more side effects. Such as the Latin adage, thousands of years old, **PRIMUM NON NOCERE**, meaning "First, do not harm", remains valid today...

However, certain medications known to deteriorate cognition temporarily are being administered: antidepressants such as fluoxetine and amitriptyline, antispasmodics with an anticholinergic role (oxybutynin), anxiolytic-hypnotics (benzodiazepine), etc.

Also, these classes of drugs can interfere with the action of antidementia symptomatic medication of acetylcholinesterase inhibitor medications type, reducing their improving action on the cognitive and sometimes behavioral state of patients diagnosed with dementia.

78. Are there other remedies in Alzheimer dementia?

Memory disorders have probably accompanied humanity since its beginning, all individuals above a certain age are probably predisposed to present such changes. On the other hand, with the research of different drugs, changes could be induced (both structural and physiological) similar to those of Alzheimer's disease on different laboratory animals. Of course, as in other illnesses, prehistoric people and those closest to our time have sought natural remedies for these events. It is known that some drugs are based on such remedies (digitalis - digoxin, quinine - quinidine).

As in all medical specialties, most herbal remedies derived from traditional Chinese medicine (ginkgo biloba, ginseng).

In the domain of cognition, the effect of ginkgo biloba extract from the leaves is already recognized in the medical field to improve cerebral circulation (ginkgo trees can live 1000 years!), medications as Tanakan or Bilobil are being currently introduced in the dementias treatment. On the other hand, the same plant has a strong antioxidant effect, a mechanism taken into account in the primary prevention of dementias.

Also, the ginseng extract is considered a "panax" – universal panacea that is good in the treatment of all illnesses. Based on the tradition of Oriental medicine, ginseng is used as a mental tonic in case of mental and/or physical fatigue in depressive states, especially in the elderly but also in memory disorders.

Also, the coconut oil is considered a panacea due to its high content of unsaturated fatty acids medium chain carbon, among which the most important lauric acid (over 50%) which metabolizes at liver level, forms ketones which are used by the brain also (as well as other organs) as an energy supplier in terms of decreasing blood flow and secondly of glucose levels.

Living in a consumer society, given the advertising for natural or synthetic products, or even containing active substances at the brain level, it must call for an increased attention when using them. Unfortunately, there are too few doctors involved in traditional medicine to guide patients towards using products with real beneficial effect on the body in general and the brain in particular.

79. What are the classes of medications used to treat dementia?

Classes of drugs involved in the treatment of dementia are inhibitors of acetylcholinesterase, antagonists of NMDA receptors, neurotrophic medication, antioxidant medication, anti-inflammatory medication and NGF (nerve growth factor) type medication. The first three classes may be included in the category of "symptomatics" while the last three can be grouped in the category of "pathophysiological possibly active medication".

Symptomatic medication, considered specific to the treatment of dementia implies action on neurotransmitters involved in memory and learning processes, acetylcholine (acetylcholinesterase inhibitors) and at the level of glutamate (NMDA receptor antagonists, or N-methyl-D-aspartate). Unfortunately, the efficacy of these treatments (i.e. improvement of cognitive capacity and daily activity of the patient) is proven (more recently) for a period of one to two years maximum and, therefore, are considered to be symptomatic. However, the long-term recommendation (including in the advanced stage of Alzheimer dementia) remains valid.

Cholinergic neurons are essential for memory. They are mainly described as neurons using acetylcholine as a neurotransmitter to convey messages, information. They provide the necessary cerebral cortex acetylcholine required for various processes, including the memorization process. This is also proven by the loss of cholinergic neurons in dementia Alzheimer's and secondarily by lowering the acetylcholine in the neural synapses. Likewise, damaging of the cholinergic tracts causes cognitive disorders. Other studies report that restoration of cholinergic synapses improves memory.

To improve the level of acetylcholine at the synapses level, many chemical agents can be used: acetylcholinesterase inhibitors, muscarinic antagonists (EC muscarinic acting on M1 receptors) and nicotinic antagonists. It is for this reason that nicotine intake by smoking has originally a role in improving the processing of information. Its negative role comes from chronic use, for periods of years or decades through the effect of toxic compounds in the cigarettes, tar in particular.

Of all agents, the inhibitors of acetylcholinesterase became the first in the treatment of dementia. Adverse reactions are of the cholinergic type, especially digestive problems (nausea, vomiting) and much rarer of the cardiac type (atrio-ventricular blocks) requiring a electrocardiographic monitoring at initiation of treatment.

Their history is long, starting with Tacrine which was decommissioned due to its hepatic toxicity, short action time (took 4 doses/day) and the necessity of managing large doses to take effect. Later donepezil and rivastigmine emerged, with positive effects in smaller doses and with fewer side effects. Later, the FDA has approved in the United States the use of galantamine also.

Donepezil has the advantage of one daily dose only, mild side effects (nausea and vomiting, as well as other agents in this class) and effectiveness in improving cognition, global status and functionality. The effective dose is 10 mg daily. The effects are quickly visible (days, weeks) but diminish progressively until about 2 years when some researchers argue that they are no longer effective. However, the general condition worsens after discontinuation of the drug and in the more advanced stages of the illness.

Rivastigmine is a pseudo-reversible acetylcholinesterase inhibitor, having butyrylcholinesterase inhibitor effect in addition, as compared to other components in its class.

Initially, the presentation has been for oral administration but required two daily doses, subsequently the formula patch emerged with a slow discharge (24 hours) going up to a daily dose of 13.3 mg. The initiation is done with a minimum dose (1.5 or 3 mg) and is increased gradually up to the maximum therapeutic dose tolerated by the patient.

Glutamate is the most important excitatory amino acid neurotransmitter at the cortical and hippocampal neurons level. Sustained increase of levels of glutamate and/or increased sensitivity to glutamate causes alteration of the neuronal homeostasis (involving calcium ions) in Alzheimer dementia and ultimately neurodegeneration. The main glutamate-activated receptor – the N-methyl-D-aspartate (NMDA) receiver is involved in the central neural mechanism responsible for learning and memory through the long term potentiation (LTP). Memantine is a non-selective antagonist voltage-dependent and with a moderate affinity for NMDA receptors. It blocks the pathological effects of increased levels of glutamate which leads to dysfunction and ultimately to neuronal death, but on the other hand, facilitates LTP process also. The daily dose of memantine is 20 mg administered in two doses with a small dose initiation – 5 mg and slow (weekly) growth up to the therapeutic dose.

The **neurotrophic medication** is the medication which improves blood flow to the brain structures, thus to the structures involved in cognition (the limbic system - Appendix 9). Although they use a lot of nerve agents (piracetam, vinpocetine, vincamine, etc.) their action is not proven by meta-analyzes (major studies), the effect of which is symptomatic at most. In medical practice however, there is a noticeable improvement in specific psychometric tests at 3 and 6 months of treatment.

A series of studies were conducted in the **possibly active pathophysiological category of medication** for the role of **the antioxidant medication** in lowering neuronal free radicals (oxidative stress seeming to play a pivotal role in the pathogenesis of Alzheimer's). Among them, the most studied were vitamin E, ginkgo biloba extract, monoamine oxidase inhibitors and less vitamin C which also has a strong antioxidant effect. The recommended doses for antioxidant effect are 1000-2000 mg/day of vitamin E, gingko biloba 80-120 mg daily and 1000 mg of vitamin C.

Gerovital emerged in the 60s, in the case of monoamine oxidase inhibitors, which is an eutrophic drug produced in Romania, and which has this secondary effect also. Gerovital was recognized at the time for its effect of prevention of aging, including the brain structures (especially at the cell membrane), with positive effects in the process of memorizing and learning new information. In my professional experience, I have found that thousands of patients who use long-term Gerovital show decreased frequency of cognitive impairments as opposed to those who for various reasons were not administered preparation. Gerovital continues to be produced today as a nutritional supplement in Romania and is very popular in many countries worldwide.

More recently, studies have been conducted for vitamin C also, which besides the antioxidant effect appears to have a lowering effect generation of β-amyloid and lowering of acetylcholinesterase (an enzyme that degrades acetylcholine and thus decreases its concentration at the neuronal synapsis.)

Regarding the anti-inflammatory medication, this would decrease the devastating effect of inflammation – caused by activation of microglia and astroglia (nerve cells with supportive but also nutritional role of the central nervous system) – on the neurons and by default on the cognitive function. Among these, the anti-inflammatory type coxibs were the most commonly used (nonsteroid anti-inflammatory medication with lower adverse gastrointestinal effects than other anti-inflammatory drugs) but the majority of studies were suspended due to thrombotic risk (bleeding, especially in the digestive system).

Last but not least, medication type "nerve growth factor" has been used for over 10 years and gaining more and more ground in both the treatment of Alzheimer's and vascular dementia. In recent years, the use of **cerebrolysin** (an extract of swine protein) in a daily dose of up to 30 ml, in a program for 10 days per month is recommended in over 40 countries around the world, except the United States where the FDA has not given consent for this treatment.

80. How frequent are the side effects of the administered medicine?

Regarding the side effects of drugs used in dementia, two things are prevalent.

The first aspect refers to adverse drug reactions in general but also in the elderly, in particular. It is said that a drug has a positive effect and 10 adverse effects. Then, medication administration must take into account the interaction between drugs. On the other hand, an elderly patient suffering from polypathology (several illnesses simultaneously) in different medical areas (heart, kidney, digestive, respiratory, oncology, etc.) results in a polypharmacy. Often, the elder patient goes through different specialty clinics and finally sums up all those recommendations without anyone considering the iatrogenesis (secondary illnesses due to the administration of drugs).

Here, the essential role of the geriatrician comes into picture, who as the internist for the elderly must comb through this stuffy scheme, considering the importance and severity of illnesses, but also the side effects and interactions of the recommended medicines.

Another important issue is to assess the renal function (creatinine clearance - a mathematical formula that takes into account the patient's age), administration of drugs being done according to it and sometimes when it comes to a fragile patient (meaning the "fragility syndrome of the elderly" – see Question 40) leading up to the administration of body weight (kg) medication dosage, just as in the pediatric service.

Do not interrupt or reduce medication without the doctor's advice!

The second issue is strictly related to side effects of specific drugs administered in dementia, most of these drugs being symptomatic (including those which treat complications or non-cognitive symptoms of the illness).

Among the most feared side effects, we should mention here:

- Acetylcholinesterase inhibitors through type cholinergic reactions cause abdominal pain, vomiting, diarrhea, as well as atrioventricular blocks, so the initiating medication is recommended to be done in a specialized clinic admissions.

- Antipsychotics of neuroleptics type (especially the "typical" ones – from the first generation) determine extrapyramidal syndrome reactions with risk of imbalance in motion (secondarily, falls with femoral fractures or head trauma), hypotension, syncope (see Question 82), leading infrequently to "malignant neuroleptic syndrome", with intense fever - body temperature over 40 degrees Celsius - with an often unfavorable evolution and leading to death in a matter of hours/days.

- Benzodiazepine-type anxiolytics emphasize the cognitive impairment, causing sleepiness, risk of falls, often paradoxical reactions such as disinhibition and agitation, requiring caution and regular monitoring of blood pressure during the day.

- Tricyclic antidepressants cause urinary retention, orthostatic hypotension leading to syncope and to falls, disorientation and confusion.

- "Nerve growth factor" medication type cause, rarely, allergic reactions, requiring skin tests prior to their administration.

Considering all these presented aspects, the conclusion is:

> Do not alter the specific treatment plan without the doctor's advice!

81. Are there currently any new medications in research phase?

If the drugs currently in use for symptomatic dementia are symptomatic, possible new medication is directed towards different segments of its pathogenic chain.

Thus there are three main research directions in development:

- Destruction or preventing of the formation of β-amyloid plaques in particular at the extracellular level, located at the synapses, and which initially prevent the transmission of information at this level
- Preventing the formation of protein tangles resulting from protein agglomeration (hyperphosphorylated tau protein) belonging to the neuronal cytoskeleton, having the transport role for neuronal metabolism nutrients
- Decreasing or annihilation of neuronal inflammatory processes observed in the pathological process of Alzheimer's disease

Regarding the specific treatment for annihilating action β-amyloid, various forms of vaccine are in research, which work on certain enzymes with role in the cleavage (α secretion) or aggregation (γ and β secretion) of these protein structures (aggregated β-amyloid that precursors the β-amyloid). Thus, these substances will stimulate either α secretion or will inhibit β and γ secretion. Intensive research in Phase II had been interrupted due to the emergence of a significant number of secondary encephalitis (18 cases per 298 patients). A new study, which takes into account the limits of previous studies, suggests an intranasal vaccine for direct action in the brain.

The treatments proposed for intervention in hyperphosphorylation of tau protein use glycogen synthase kinase 3b-inhibitors (GSK -3b) and Cyclin-dependent kinase 5 (CDK -5).

Recently, in 2014 Jian Xu and Paul Lombroso reported the discovery of a new class of inhibitory drugs - TC 2153 which action the striatal - enriched protein tyrosine phosphatase (STEP) and regulate synaptic glutamate receptor, involved learning and memory.

Given the current state of research in this field, many experts are hoping to discover soon at least one drug to treat the illness unless it is complex therapy, as in the case for cancer or the human immunodeficiency syndrome.

82. What are the complications of an antipsychotic treatment and what should we do?

Initially, typical neuroleptics were used during the course of antipsychotic treatment evolution and subsequently to reduce the atypical side effects (18/100 patients receiving neuroleptic therapy).

The characteristics of first-generation antipsychotics therapy (typical neuroleptics):

- Haloperidol was originally used as an antipsychotic therapy in dementia
- Low antipsychotic potential (thioridazine e.g., Chlorpromazine) having anticholinergic, sedative and hypotensive properties
- Increased potential of walking troubles, causing extrapyramidal side effects more frequently

The characteristics of the second generation of antipsychotic therapy (atypical neuroleptics):

- Antipsychotic effects much improved over the previous generation
- It determines greatly reduced side effects relative to typical neuroleptics:

  - Cognitive impairment.

  - Hypotension.

- Extrapyramidal side effects with walking difficulties lower than first class.

- Neuroleptic malignant syndrome, hyperthermia (40 degrees Celsius), very rarely.

The most frequently used antipsychotics are risperidone, quetiapine, olanzapine. Given the significant side effects of this class of drugs, even for atypical neuroleptics, my recommendation is that the administration be done strictly under the specialist guidance, the initiation of therapy would be desirable to be done in a hospital environment for effective supervision of adverse reactions, as well as minimal useful dosage for long-term treatment. In addition, in terms of behavioral disorders each patient behaves differently and therefore requires an individual approach.

> If their use is unavoidable, then the atypical antipsychotics are the least harmful, but the loading dose should be low, gradually increasing, and once the desired effect is reached, the daily dose should be reduced to the minimum effective limit.

83. How should we act if the patient is agitated or even violent?

There are two distinct categories of intervention in psychotic episodes characterized by agitation, hallucinations (usually visual), ideas of persecution or harm, and sometimes even verbal and physical violence.

The first refers to non-pharmacological measures to be initiated as soon as a change in patient behavior is being noticed. The main measure is psychotherapy, and considering that most often around the patient there is no psychologist available, that patient caregivers must know how to communicate with them. Caregivers should receive detailed advice about the illness in general and about "crisis" events, whereby the patient may harm others or himself. They must know the techniques of communication with the patient.

Communication is of three types: verbal, non-verbal and para-verbal. If the apparent verbal communication is the most important (spoken language) in reality non-verbal communication, namely "body language" hand, facial or body signs, are means by which the "bridge" can be achieved connecting with a patient who has an impoverished language, as it is the case of a patient with dementia behavioral disorders.

The specialists make some recommendations for caregivers of patients in order to avoid or minimize such problems:

- Impose on the patient an active program and a routine during the day. The afternoon nap should not exceed one hour.
- Organize a one dish dinner without stimulants (alcohol, cola). Lunch compensation must be plentiful and rich in protein.
- Limit the emergence of new events in the evening (family visit or some friends, noise).
- Set a pleasant and safe patient bedroom (bed position near the door, waking light, windows with locks, etc.).

However, if problems arise, the caregiver must act calmly, not to forbid the patient from walking (but to only accompany them), to permanently ensure that everything is alright without engaging in arguments (the carer's vocabulary must not contain the word NO and negations in general).

In case of extreme agitation, the patient will be restrained for a limited period, with special straps that do not cause injuries or trauma.

A second type of intervention is the use of pharmacological measures consisting of antipsychotic medication administration (see Question 82) and sedative-hypnotic (benzodiazepines have reduced side effects on the cardiac patients).

We draw attention once again that these pharmacological measures can not be taken unless a specialist recommends them.

84. What type of care should be given in the terminal phase?

Firstly, we must define the terminal dementia stage (mostly corresponding to class 7 on the Reisberg scale), the patient has a severe deterioration of their intellectual functions, with serious damage to voluntary activities, most often incontinence both for urine and faeces. Finally, the patient in the terminal phase just maintains archaic reflexes (grip and suction reflexes).

From the beginning, we need to pay attention to three important sides of the issue.

The first would be the ethical one, which establishes until what moment care is to be provided to the terminal patient. Is anyone in a position to stop this treatment when it becomes obvious that the patient no longer has any benefits from the treatment, but, on the contrary, complications which mean nothing but pain and suffering? It is a known fact that there are countries which apply euthanasia in these situations. Some of these countries allow for this option even in the stage when the patient still has discernment. Depending on the culture and religion of each nation this solution may or may not be optimal, on one major condition: to be legalized!

A second, but no less important question, is how to determine the location where this care should take place. From the start, the importance of the collaboration of the family with the team of specialists involved in treating and caring for patients must be made clear, regardless of whether care takes place at the patient's home or in an institutional environment (long term care center, nursing home, center for palliative care). This decision must take into account, unfortunately, socioeconomic factors, in some cases, to the detriment of the medical factors. Often, in many countries, care services at home, which would be recommended in the first instance, in the absence of behavioral troubles, can not be sustained by the state, so families need to move to a more or less specialized care center, according to their financial possibilities.

A third side, certainly the most important, concerns providing medical and professional care when the patient remains in the family. The family must have the support of health professionals who recommend and supervise patient's care (correct administration of food and hydration, physical therapy procedures to prevent bedsores, hygiene rules, etc.).

The decision to institutionalize a patient with dementia is taken by the family and a multidisciplinary team, considering the following factors:

1. Severe impact on the patient's daily activity, as assessed by ADL (Appendix 10) and IADL (Appendix 11), regardless of the degree of cognitive impairment.

2. Severe behavioral disorders ("admission crisis").

3. Family environment, either inadequate or unable of providing quality care.

4. Costs and resources – community or private institutionalization, as applicable.

5. Family structure.

> The main characteristics of dementia which require initiation of care in specialized centers are the severity of functional impairment and the presence of behavioral disorders. Cognitive impairment is less important than the first two!

Providing long-term care for patients with dementia varies from one country to another.

The decision to place a relative in a long-term institution is difficult and brings along feelings of guilt and pain. On the other hand, there are positive aspects such as the treatment of insomnia and behavioral disturbances, with effect on improving the quality of life which counterbalances in favor of institutionalization.

There is a correlation between the specific institutional expenditures and the care needs of the people affected by dementia in the northern countries and Western Europe, the former with higher levels of formal care than the latter. Mediterranean countries and the countries of Central and Southern Europe show a low correlation of the two (expenses/needs). In comparison, the correlation dynamics trends are linear, unstable and unclear.

Any project to create a care institution dedicated to patients with dementia is a compromise, on one hand between the achievement of conditions (short or long term) similar to a family environment and the necessity of providing quality medical services and on the other hand, between what is desired and what is achievable on affordable costs/prices.

Conversely, the good functioning of such an institution care includes providing a regular medical control, proper handling of behavioral disorders (including psychological counseling) and a plan of activities tailored to each patient.

85. Should drug therapy be discontinued in the terminal phase?

The answer to this question is absolutely not! There are some drugs with the indication to be interrupted (according to some authors), such as acetylcholinesterase inhibitors and even NMDA receptor antagonists, considering that at this stage they would not have any effect. From medical practice, I have seen that the discontinuation of anti-dementia medication however, be it symptomatic as the two classes mentioned above, accelerates the end of the illness.

Despite a serious health condition, the patient who is in the terminal phase of dementia is considered to be conscious and, naturally, must be given the opportunity to a dignified life until the end. Often, at the end of this evolution of such a patient, we found (puzzlingly sometimes) that the pacient may have an inexplicable moment of lucidity in which they even recognize their family and are able to say farewell to them!

Thus, the support fluid (fluid intake), medications for heart pathology, nutritional support (enteral or parenteral) must accompany the patient to the end of their life.

86. Is institutionalization compulsory in the terminal phase?

It is obvious that on condition that all support and medical care means can be provided, it would be ideal for the patient to live their last moments of life in the family.

However, given that most times these professional services can not be met at home, the patient's doctor must explain to the family why the patient can be better cared for and treated in a specialized environment. Unfortunately, worldwide, there is a lack of such places in hospitals (even in the private sector).

87. How should we behave around a terminal patient?

As I stated in a previous question (see Question 85), the patient is conscious and must be treated with dignity. Even if sometimes the patient does not understand spoken language, they are good receivers for sign messages (non-verbal communication, see Question 83), through affection and spiritual closeness.

In order to increase the patient's comfort level, nursing preparation and hygiene should be done gently and patiently, trying to reduce pain as much as possible and to prevent the risk of complications which can be fatal either directly or through the complications they can cause (swallowing disorders, bedsores).

Death in degenerative dementias is inevitable, regardless of the neurodegeneration type, with no known cure at this time. This occurs through a complication - pneumonia, asphyxiation by swallowing disorders, severe vascular events (stroke – most commonly, acute myocardial infarction – rare).

88. Do all patients reach the stage of bed confinement?

This is a question which worries equally the patient diagnosed with dementia as well as their caregivers. Definitely not, the situation is similar to any elderly, just that in patients with dementia this situation is more common.

It has to be said that depending on coexisting pathology (cardiac or neurological illnesses, cancer, etc.), the patient may or may not reach the stage of confinement in bed.

What is more important in order to avoid such a situation, is the way the patient with dementia is cared for and treated, this depending on whether and how long the patient remains bedridden. Thus, a good physiotherapy (neurological recovery) and cognitive programme may delay this phenomenon, so as the period to be as short as possible.

89. What are the complications of bed confinement?

Complications of confinement to bed are inevitable, regardless of the level of care for the patient.

Weight loss occurs during this evolution, not only by inadequate diets but especially by a decrease in the intestinal absorption. In the final stage, despite parenteral administration (intravenous) with a nutrient solution, cachexia appears (very pronounced weight loss) with increased risk of decubitus (trophic lesions in the skin) at pressure areas (especially sacral area).

Severe complications of bed confinement are pneumonia, vascular accidents (stroke or myocardial infarction), and finally acute cardio-respiratory failure.

Pneumonia is in most cases a pneumonia stasis (patient position should be changed every 2 hours and patted on their back at least twice daily), with his own germs, which, due to the severe decrease of immunity, become pathogenic, or as a second possibility, an aspiration pneumonia, through aspiration of gastric juice or more or less digested food.

Vascular events relate mainly to either a stroke (most commonly in vascular dementia than Alzheimer dementia) or an acute myocardial infarction.

Finally, the cardiopulmonary arrest sets-in, which in most countries is non-recoverable, considering that it has set in naturally during the illness evolution and the benefits of "recovering" the patient albeit of lack of cure, would be just an illusion.

90. Is there a diet which protects against Alzheimer's disease?

Of all the dietary proposals which would protect a person against memory illnesses, the most famous is the Mediterranean diet.

The Mediterranean diet is based on whole grains, vegetables, fruits, fish, cheese products, yogurt or fermented milk and olive oil, a daily glass of red wine being also mentioned in this diet. The Mediterranean diet contains such significant quantities of beta - carotene, vitamin C, tocopherols and tocotrienols (i.e., vitamin E), polyphenols, and essential minerals (selenium, magnesium, zinc, iron, calcium).

The antioxidant is the main effect of the Mediterranean diet. This would block the emergence of "bad" cholesterol and its deposit onto the blood vessels in the form of plates (atheroma), which cause their narrowing and eventually blockage, both in healthy people and diabetics. Also, for patients who are overweight (body mass index, BMI > 30) this type of diet lowers total cholesterol by about 13% and systolic blood pressure by 3 mmHg. The classification of the nutritional status according to the Body Mass Index is highlighted in Appendix 11.

Studies which have compared the Mediterranean diet with the typical American diet have shown that the former significantly prolongs survival time of patients already diagnosed with Alzheimer dementia. Researchers followed 192 Alzheimer's patients over a period of 4 years. Patients who had a diet similar to the Mediterranean diet lived 1.3 years longer than those who had a typical American diet. According to these studies, those who strictly followed the Mediterranean diet lived exactly four years longer.

Other studies have shown that the diet specific to the Mediterranean coast decreases the risk of heart attack nine times on one hand, but also reduces the risk of osteoporosis and the bone fracture risk as a secondary effect.

Also, there are plenty of studies (conducted by reputed physicians and researchers) which take into account its positive effects on cognition - sometimes by changes in the senile cerebral plaques or neurofibrillary tangles of tau protein - of the nutritional supplements added to the daily diet (cinnamon, curry, coffee or cacoa).

Last but not least, I would like to tell you something about the antiinflammatory diet. It's well-known that chronic inflammation is the basis of all chronic diseases in which we include some heart diseases, cancers and also neurodegenerative diseases, including Alzheimer's disease. Inflammation can be triggered by various external factors among which the most important in our times are stress, smoking and a diet rich in preservatives, food colorings or metals. This is the reason why an antiinlammatory diet seems adequate in Alzheimer dementia and in other types of dementia.

Among the proinflamatory diets, we mention those that are based on white flour, sugar and also sweeteners, fried foods, red meat and processed foods, hydrogenated fats, etc. Instead, antiinflammatory foods are fresh fruits, raw vegetables, legumes, oleaginous seeds, fish and whole grains.

91. *How do we assess the nutritional status of patients with dementia?*

The assessment of the nutritional state, as part of the standard geriatric evaluation of the patient with the diagnosis of dementia involves the following antropometric indices:

• weight,

• height,

• Body Mass Index (BMI = Weight (kg)/Height^2 (cm^2)) is more relevant than the direct correlation of wieght with height, especially in the elderly.

The classification of nutritional status on the elderly is made according to the body mass index (see Appendix 10).

Mini Nutritional Assessment (MNA) is a practical method which allows a quick and simple assessment of the elderly at risk of malnutrition, in order to allow intervention at the optimum time in terms of nutrition, without the need of a specialized team of nutritionists. MNA is a rapid method for assessing nutritional status which has been validated in many countries, because of its ease of performing, effectiveness of the obtained data, but especially due to the fact that we can have a common language assessment, at last.

The integration of this geriatric assessment test helps the practitioner in early detection of people at risk of malnutrition and to act optimally to the patient's benefit through intervention about their nutrition and to investigate the causes of this nutritional disorder.

The MNA test consists of:

• Anthropometric measurements: weight, height, skin fold, arm circumference, calf circumference.

- Global Assessment: six questions about lifestyle, medications, mobility

- Questionnaire on diet: eight questions about the number of daily meals, food intake, liquid, feeding autonomy

- Subjective appreciation: self-perception of health.

- The goal of each stage is to assess elderly patients:

- Normal (proper nutrition status),
- Borderline (risk of malnutrition),
- Malnourished.

Maximum score = 30

MNA classifies the elderly into three categories based on the 30 points on the scale:

- 24-30 = Normal.

- At risk of malnutrition from 17 to 23.5.

- <17 = malnourished.

92. What are the investigations in the nutritional status evaluation of Alzheimer's?

The investigations used in evaluating nutritional status of patients with dementia are biological samples (blood, urine), skin tests and imaging (radiography, ultrasound, CT scans).

Biological samples:

In plasma:

- Complete blood count: hematocrit, hemoglobin, red cell indices, total leukocyte count, differential white blood count, platelets.
- Plasma proteins: albumin, globulin, prealbumina, transferrin.
- Urea, creatinine, uric acid.
- Plasma Lipids: cholesterol (LDL cholesterol, HDL cholesterol), triglycerides.
- Serum ionogram: sodium, potassium, chloride, calcium, magnesium, bicarbonate, phosphate.
- Vitamins: vitamin A, vitamin E, vitamin D3, vitamin K, vitamin C, folate, vitamin B12.

In urine:

- Thiamin, riboflavin, N-methylnicotinamide.

- Minerals: iron, zinc, copper, manganese.

- Urea, creatinine, uric acid, hydroxyproline.

Skin tests – used to assess the cell-mediated immunity (the index of late hypersensitivity quantifies the skin induration obtained through the skin test, on common antigens as those derived from Candida or Trichophyton), characteristic of malnutrition being an induration grade 0<0, 5 cm (normal = 0,5-0,9 cm gr 1, w 2>1 cm).

Imaging samples are the thoracic X-rays used to assess the cardiopulmonary function, bone radiographs to assess bone density, gastrointestinal barium tract radiography, ultrasound, CT and MRI for evidence of soft tissues.

93. *What is the proper nutrition in Alzheimer dementia?*

In a recent search on the internet, we have found that more than half of dementia topics are dedicated to illness specific nutrition. It shows both its role in the surveillance plan as well as its importance granted especially by family and the population at large.

On the other hand, in a prestigious medical database, also on the internet, the report is completely disproportionate. From over 130,000 scientific articles devoted to dementia only about 1,500 (about 1%!) refer to an adequate nutrition in Alzheimer's disease. This shows how much we have to continue insisting on this important facet of the illness to be addressed in the studies and research accomplished by specialists.

Intervention in nutrition of patients with dementia must be triggered if:

1. Patient weight decreased in the last 3-6 months

or if

2. More than 2 criteria are met:

a. MNA score <17

b. The serum albumin <35 g/L

c. Decreased food intake for three days in a row

A few general considerations resulting from literature, and especially from medical practice:

- The nutritional status should be assessed even at the stage of dementia diagnosis.
- The nutritional evaluation includes at least weighing and carrying out an evaluation through the Mini Nutritional Assessment (MNA), using the caregivers' or family's help.
- The patient with dementia will be absolutely weighed at the specialist consultation.
- A weight loss of more than 2 kg weight compared to known weight, or anorexia (lack of appetite to eat) should alert the family to request a nutritional evaluation by a specialist.
- Weight loss is a common complication of Alzheimer dementia in about 40% of patients, regardless of the illness stage.
- Malnutrition contributes to overall health alteration, by the frequent occurrence of complications (particularly, infections through immunity deterioration), but also to the effect on the degree of independence. It requires a rapid and appropriate response.

- In the geriatric population, a loss of >4% of body weight per year is considered an independent factor for morbidity and mortality.
- Losing weight can be of 2 types: a rapid loss in a few months or a moderate weight loss over the evolution of dementia.
- It is considered that a weight loss of 4% or more over the last 3-6 months require nutritional program initiation.
- An anorexic patient or under treatment with acetylcholinesterase inhibitor requires an assessment of another cause, other than the treatment of choice for the illness.
- Investigation of reversible medical or social causes, increased calories intake/protein (or more oral dietary supplements) and physical activity are the primary measures in the nutritional management.
- Stressful medical situations such as severe infections or surgeries require adequate nutritional support.
- "The gold standard" in nutritional evaluation is the use of the blood-biomarkers (see Question 92).
- With the standardization of nutritional biomarkers, interactive studies be can initiated using their combinations to

see how they can influence chronic illnesses, including Alzheimer dementia.

- A high amount of saturated fats cause amyloidosis type Alzheimer dementia, while the calories restriction by reducing carbohydrate intake can prevent it.
- Depressive patients with hallucinations and behavioral disorders are more exposed to undernutrition than subjects without these symptoms.
- A proper assessment of nutritional status can prevent and treat problems related to nutrition even for the patient who is not institutionalized.

Understanding of nutritional status is mandatory even from the diagnostic stage of the illness. Since 2001 there have been a number of epidemiological studies which have researched the association between cognition and nutrition (particularly fatty acids, antioxidants such as vitamins C, A, E and polyphenols). Other studies have been trying to identify the role of various nutrients, the influence of genetic factors and lifestyle on brain aging and dementia.

Both Alzheimer dementia and vascular dementia – which share in principle, the same risk factors (vascular risk factors are common) - should target some recommendations related to nutrition in primary prevention.

Cognitive impairment correlates with nutritional status: the patient with cognitive impairment has a better MNA score than patient diagnosed with dementia. On the other hand, there are studies which show a linear relationship between malnutrition and rapid drop in cognitive scores (a decrease in MMSE >3 points in one year). Also, malnourished patients show a rapid worsening of the illness, but paradoxically have the best response to treatment with acetylcholinesterase inhibitors.

Other studies show that patients with Alzheimer dementia have an increased level of oxidative stress biomarkers; consequently, their nutritional intervention must increase plasma antioxidant levels and decrease the oxidative stress. In a prospective study over a six year period, on a total of 3700 participants in the "Chicago Health and Age Project", the increased consumption of fruits and vegetables was associated with slowed cognitive decline, after correction for age, sex, race and education, cardiovascular conditions and present risk factors.

The Mediterranean diet demonstrates that nutritional intervention has great potential to positively influence the evolution of dementia.

Patients at risk should put into practice some recommendations:

- consume a diet rich in fish, nuts, seeds, olives and olive oil;
- limit consumption of foods and drinks which affect the balance between insulin and glucose serum (especially fine sweets - sugar, confectionery products);
- follow, if possible, a Mediterranean-type diet;
- see a specialist as soon as they or their family notice weight loss, having the doctor determine whether diet changes are needed.

> The first goal of nutritional support is to maintain if not increase the patient's quality of life!

Other objectives to observe:

- ensure the necessary protein, energy and micronutrients and vitamins intake;
- maintain or improve nutritional status;

- maintain and improve functionality, activities and the overall recovery;
- reduce mortality and morbidity.

94. How is proper hydration achieved for a patient with dementia?

It is known that a patient with dementia has an increased degree of risk to dehydrate as the stage of the illness is more advanced. The reasons are manifold and multiply along with the evolution of the illness:

- administration of diuretics (Antihypertensive medication which increases diuresis (liquid elimination through urine));
- alcohol and caffeine consumption;
- decrease of the sensation of thirst (affecting the thirst centre located in the brain, in dementia);
- deglutition disorders cause chocking fear for both the patient and caregiver, especially with liquids;
- deficiencies of verbal communication needs – including the need for hydration;
- the existence of intestinal transit disorders – diarrhoea, vomiting - with the derived loss of fluid (and minerals);

- occurrence of urinary incontinence – determines reduction in voluntary ingestion (intake) of water.
- inadequate fluid intake administered to the patient by the caregiver through lack of knowledge or negligence.

Dehydration is caused by the imbalance in body fluid intake/loss, unfavorable to the intake (less liquid ingested). Liquids have a vital role in the transport of nutrients and oxygen (in the blood) to all cells in the body, maintaining the organs and the body in a condition of optimal functionality, including the prevention of constipation and regulating body temperature.

The amount of water in the body varies depending on age and gender. It varies between 50-75% in different organs and tissues of the body (73% in the brain). Mental and physical performance diminishes even with a 2-3% decrease of the total water quantity. That is why a patient with dementia who is dehydrated presents a stronger cognitive impairment and a confusion state. Other symptoms which occur in dehydration can be: the sensation of "dry mouth", rarely "tongue burns", fatigue, lethargy, headaches, dizziness, tachypnea (rapid breathing).

As a result, the question of how much water does a patient with dementia need to take on a daily basis? There is a fairly large variability of proposals from professionals, but, in any case, one should be mindfull of the patient's altering health state (heart illness, kidney illness, increased body temperature).

For a mild dehydration, a moderate additional fluid ingestion is sufficient, knowing that an adult person must take in 2-2.5 liters of liquids daily (this can be calculated according to body weight, about 30 ml/kg bw/day). Water is not the only source, to achieve an adequate intake of fluids and non-carbonated sweet liquids such as fruit juices, fruits that contain large amounts of water (watermelons, grapes, cucumbers, lettuce, tomatoes, etc.), dairy (milk, yogurt), soups and even semi-solid preparations can also be used.

If the doctor identifies a more important dehydration (presence of specific signs, such as persistent skin fold), frequent in advanced forms of dementia, this requires parenteral (intravenous) administration of fluids chosen according to some constant blood biochemical analysis results (urea, creatinine, natremia, potassemia, blood sugar). Glucozate, hydrosaline, Ringer solutions will be used, but only with the specialist's advice.

Tips for administering fluids to patients with dementia:

• include juicy fruits and vegetables in one's daily diet (besides the fluid intake they also provide fiber needs for a proper digestion)

• offer particularly fluids preferred by the patient (juice, yogurts, soups)

• help or supervise patients with deglutition disorders

• encourage the patient to ingest liquids

• persevere in adminstering fluids in small/moderate quantities at short intervals

95. Can dementia be cured with a natural treatment?

As in most incurable diseases different "quacks" appear claiming that they can treat and even cure them... I will not dwell much on this subject, I just want to warn those whom, because of emotional factors triggered when first faced with such a diagnosis, resort to other "natural methods" of treatment, trumpeted by excessive advertising especially promoted on the internet for fabulous earnings (for the producers!).

However, we do not deny the role of plants or extracts of those plants which have a positive effect especially on illness-specific symptoms of memory (see Question 78). Of these gingko remains the most studied extract with proven neurotrophic effect.

We insist that any so-called natural treatment be certified by the specialist, who will verify the composition of these products, their possible positive effect, but especially the side effects of different compounds thereof.

96. *Is the early diagnosis of Alzheimer's disease useful and ethical?*

We are still at the beginning of the debate on this subject.

Firstly, we can say that it is useful to quickly get knowledge diagnosis of possible Alzheimer's illness (also acknowledging the presence of some genetic markers) considering the new data on prevention, taking into account the influence of risk factors (vascular, stress, traumatic, smoking, etc.) (see Questions 25-29, 31) and the possible presence of reversible dementia which can be countered if early intervention is initiated (curative treatment) (see Question 56).

In this regard, we must consider other examples, which in turn have given justice to those who proposed them! For example, aggressive anti-smoking campaign displayed on cigarette packs in Western countries, which has been successful and decreased the number of smokers.

In this context, awareness of diagnosis by the subject becomes ethically valid, even in the pre-dementia stage in which either there are no symptoms or changes in cognitive function are insufficient to affect daily activity, as it happens in Alzheimer dementia. Of course, the psychological counseling and the involvement of a specialist to explain all possible sides of dementia appearance are mandatory, so the patient and their family take the best long-term decisions.

97. *Should we be afraid of dementia?*

Although this question, as the next two, refers to the emotional rather than the medical and philosophical states, we considered necessary in the light of experience gained over so many years, to try to answer such questions. Certainly, there is a high degree of subjectivity, but maybe it is more important to respond with the soul than with the mind in such debates.

As I previously stated, during my work in this area, which I often consider rather delicate than complicated, I have experienced this feeling of fear which concerned both the patient at the start of this journey, as well as the family. I always tell my patients and their families that fear is a natural human feeling which is part of our human development. So consequently, we must not repress this fear but we understand it, to look for explanations and answers to our problems. Thus, good knowledge of the illness and its progression, will result with time in reduced feelings of fear which will be replaced by the desire of deep feeling for the time left.

Rediscovering hobbies (painting, reading, gardening, etc.) and spiritual, religious life, and taking trips which they always wanted, time spent with the family, are all values that turn the feeling of fear into spiritual fulfillment.

Not infrequently, the loss of certain skills can be the first step toward acquiring skills which can create entirely new experiences, sometimes amazing, both for the patient and family...

98. Can we accept the harsh reality of a dementia diagnosis?

The most difficult for the family and the patient is accepting this illness and, implicitly, its unfavorable evolution. The role of the specialist, especially the psychologist's, is to make a ruthless diagnosis in a natural step in our journey between two unknown worlds, one before birth and the other after death. The only way forward is reconciliation with themselves on the path of faith which brings a feeling of accomplishment in the human soul. Thus, for the last part of their life, they can focus on themselves and their families performing good deeds, by prioritizing the values to leave for the generations to follow.

Among the thousands of patients I have had so far, I saw people reconciled with their fate and unlike those with rapidly evolving terminal illnesses (such as some forms of cancer), patients with dementia have time to reflect on how they will leave this world...

When, unfortunately, the patient goes through the terminal phase of the illness, they remind their family about Jesus' sacrifice for the good of His peers, and they try to make them understand that sometimes we are called to present our oblation to God.

99. *Can we live through this illness with dignity?*

The answer is certainly yes! It depends on the doctor and their team to explain all the unknowns of this illness, to achieve a long-term communication with both the patient and their family.

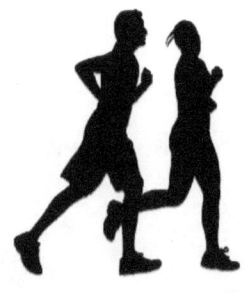

Often, almost paradoxically, patients with Alzheimer dementia possess an unbeatable health (I've seen patients who survived after they wandered barefoot outisde in the winter!) so that, from the time of diagnosis until the end of the illness, they can sometimes go through more than a decade of life with proper care and treatment.

Thus, identifying this diagnostic, has to be but a signal that the Latin saying "Carpe diem" must be applied immediately for a long and beautiful life...

100. What are the myths and misconceptions about Alzheimer's disease?

<u>Alzheimer's disease does not exist, impaired cognition is something that occurs naturally with aging...</u>

Perhaps the most important myth is that Alzheimer's disease is something natural in the general process of aging, representing a normal brain damage. It is true that this physiological process called aging causes a cognitive dysfunction more pronounced with age, secondary to the decrease in the number of neurons and synapses between them in the complex structures of the brain, but will not always evolve into dementia, as I defined it from the start (see Question 2), when the memory and thinking deficit are sufficient to cause an important functional inability of the body.

Unfortunately, this myth has long circulated among physicians; however, current evidence makes it so that it is only accepted by a reduced population with a reduced level of education.

Once diagnosed, dementia is an incurable disease..

This myth is busted including throughout this guide (see Question 52) through the evidence of those existing reversible dementia types which – as I have shown before – are curable. It is very important that the specialist takes into account these types of dementia when making differential diagnosis and not fall into the trap of the first diagnosis, often unsustainable, of Alzheimer dementia. Even in this book, in order to popularize it, we gave the generic name of "Alzheimer's" to everything which involves cognitive pathology, bringing – throughout this book – countless proofs for a multitude of causes and types of dementia.

The patient's and family's fear of Alzheimer dementia (sometimes of the "Alzheimer's" word itself) delays the diagnostics and implicitly the treatment of dementia.

The stigma associated with loss of lucidity and independence prevents families and patients from accepting the possibility of existence of this illness, often seeing a specialist when it is already late, when dementia is already in a medium or severe stage. This is in the case for patients with a high educational level (university studies, outstanding professional skills) due to their high compensation capacity of the cognitive impairment and sometimes of the functional deficit that is sometimes associated to a high degree of disimulation (deficit masking).

It is the role of the general practitioner but also of the family members with medical training to guide the patient immediately to a physician even in the case of minor problems related to cognitive processes (not just memory but lack of attention, faulty reasoning) or behavioral issues (suddenly emerging personality disorders, ideas of prejudice and/or persecution, apathy, sadness).

If I have "memory problems", I will definitely have "Alzheimer's"!

This myth also must be dispelled by the specialist through explaining that not everyone with "memory problems" will become a patient with dementia. (Questions 34 and 35). This fear also creates undue concerns to the concerned person, and the reverse reaction of not seeing a specialist. This is more common among those who have had at least one family member with the illness, and memory who unfortunately, do not know the low level of genetically transmitted illness (see Question 18).

If I have cortical atrophy, I will definitely have "Alzheimer's"!

It is a proven fact that not all patients with dementia have cortical atrophy (highlighted in imaging examinations, see Question 24), as not all patients with brain atrophy will have dementia. Besides, at old ages the cerebral atrophy is present, without necessarily causing severe cognitive impairment or dementia.

Any patient with "Alzheimer's" will someday become agitated or aggressive...

This is also a misconception with no axiomatic value. Even those patients with aggression and agitation "potential", through early initiation of pharmacological (anxiolytics, antipsychotics) or non-pharmacological measures (psychotherapy), will have a smooth evolution of the illness without undesirable incidents (see Question 83).

On the other hand, by understanding the illness, caregivers can adapt their approach and methods of communication so as to prevent most often the negative behavior of the patient.

Patients with dementia can not enjoy their activities and their quality of life is always low!

Another misconception that is proven wrong by the reality! Patients with dementia can have an active and wonderful life, until the approach of the final stage of the illness. Early diagnosis (see Question 37) and initiating specific medication sooner can greatly help in this regard. Keeping a mentally and physically optimal tone, constant explanation of the emerging symptoms by the specialist, establishing a team consisting of patient-family-professionals are also very important in achieving this major goal.

Later, in terminal phase, respecting the rights and dignity of the patient in a friendly environment can bring them much love which they can feel until the end of their life.

101. **Are there miracles in Alzheimer's disease?**

I will try as much as possible to answer this question – instead of a rhetorical epilogue... But how could I answer such a question, asking you my reader in turn: "Why should we not believe in miracles when one of the most implausible "situations", namely that the universe is infinite, has an axiom value?

For those familiar with Alzheimer's disease, it is not news that as a number of patients in advanced forms of neurodegenerative dementia considered irreversible, woke up one day as if nothing special happened in life, more lucid and more present than many of us without cognitive impairments... Personally, in my lenghty experience in the field, I met with such examples, whose developments if not miraculous at least spectacular, could not be explained by anyone or anything.

I will only present two more relevant cases.

The first happened when I was still a "novice" in treating the illness and the miracle was when a patient in a severe form of the illness, score 6 scale Reisberg (Appendix 6), looking up one morning in the mirror, was shocked to see how she looked like. She immediately requested her family to come and pick her up, claiming that there is nothing wrong with her and she had never been ill. So far nothing new, a situation frequent in this illness type... But when her daughter came, the patient - using language that she had stopped using many years before because of neurocognitive advanced illness, - provided logical reasons for which she considered inappropriate a longer hospital stay... During this period of almost 2 days, of maximum coherence and lucidity, the patient showed complete recovery to a reasoning and intelligence characteristic to a person with a high educational level. And then, as if nothing had happened, after a few days, when the patient did not receive specific illness medication (at the request of the family), her cognitive and general status returned to previous level, as brutal as the modifications which had originally appeared, of a severe deterioration in terminal dementia.

The second case, more shocking than the first, was an octogenarian patient diagnosed with mixed dementia in a severe form (marked global cerebral atrophy and cerebral lacunar state at the brain tomography examination) brought for hospitalization because of severe behavioral changes (psychomotor agitation, sun-downing phenomenon, verbal and physical violence) and abnormal walking (movement difficulty, with bilateral support and broad support base). During hospitalization, we remedied existing sleep disorders (nycthemeral rate recovery – i.e. alternating normal wakefulness and sleep) and partially the behavioral disorders, while from cognitive and functional perspectives (MMSE = 0, ADL = 0/6) (see Question 59) there was no improvement during the two weeks elapsed, until the appearance of the "miracle".

After a severe febrile syndrome, which occurred during a night in which administration of anti-pyretic and antibiotic medication with broad-spectrum were made with some delay (a few hours) due to the onset of night, there was a spectacular evolution of the general condition and cognitive impairment of the patient. The next day, the patient woke up, left the bed on his own and came to the guard doctor's office with a firm step and mildly confused, not knowing where he was. Upon receiving the clarifications, he asked for the family to come, listing in great detail the members and their history. Referring to his previous state of health, the patient could recall that he was perfectly healthy and that he was doing housework, not recalling anything about the memory disorder.

The patient - even after his family's arrival - accepted to remain in the hospital and continue treatment and his general condition and cognitive corresponding to a person without memory disorders and disabilities (patient walking without support), were paradoxically maintained intact for 2 weeks, the only change in the patient's treatment was an antibiotic with broad spectrum. During this period the patient was lucid, calm and cooperative, had a restful sleep and was hydrated and fed normally (MMSE = 20 – corresponding to his educational level, ADL = 6/6). Later, over 30 days, the patient developed slowly and progressively into the previous state, both in terms of intellectual functions, but also locomotory, i.e. severe phase of a mixed dementia.

Following such cases, *two key questions emerge*:

1. *What are the causes (or cause) for these radical and complex changes in the evolution of such patients during the final stages of the illness?*
2. *Once identified can they be reproduced on a large scale to practically determine the cure for the illness?*

Work hypotheses:

1. *The existence of such (rare) cases demonstrates that the reversibility even in advanced stages of the illness is possible.*
2. *The relatively long duration of the reversibility (two weeks in the second case presented here) supports*

the possibility to sustain it long-term, possibly permanent, equivalent to curing the illness.

3. The possibility of a complete reversibility of the cognitive impairment shows that severe cortical atrophy and even the presence of the lacunar stroke in the second case are not essential in the evolution of the illness (in fact, the cortical atrophy has removed from the diagnostic criteria for dementia a long time ago).

Possible interpretations:

3. Certain conditions of the internal, humoral environment, cause changes in certain neurotransmitters (known or unknown) which activate in alternate ways (new synapses) the remaining neurons which in turn can completely reconstruct their neurocognitive and neuromotor status, probably based on the functional reserve (see question 39).

4. Hyperthermia can be a physical process which can function as a powerful factor (yet uninvestigated) as an altering, discharging factor of neurotransmitters which can be of an inflammatory or other nature, which can reverse the degenerative neurocognitive process up to curing it.

5. The treatment with certain antibiotics can trigger a reconstructive chain which causes partial or total reversibility of intellectual deficiencies (including cognitive), a hypothesis already studied in different research laboratories worldwide.

Through this relatively brief presentation, *I would like to trigger an alarm signal for the scientific world concerning a mandatory introduction in fundamental research of this hypothesis – highly feasible in my view, and then later sporadically evident in my medical practice - that the hyperthermia could play a fundamental role in the neurodegenerative process reversibility, even in its very advanced stages (see the second case presented above) and maintaining this "neurocognitive wellness" would be the next goal and would be the equivalent to curing this illness.*

Epilogue

The present book emerged from the desire to help those who are interested in understanding cognitive pathology (Alzheimer's, but also other forms of dementia) both at a scientific level (without making complex descriptions used in specialty books) and at a moral and human level. In my medical practice I have encountered most of the time confused families, even outraged by the situation, sometimes truly bizarre, in which the patient appeared to be normal, with an elevated language and in many cases with a coherent thinking, while the doctors were supporting the presence of the disease. Therefore, the most important thing appeared to be explaining, in a warm way, close to the family, but also to the patient, when the disease was not so advanced, what this diagnosis involves and what they must do in order to be able to go through the phases that follow as smoothly and accepting as possible.

Likewise, I was asked countless times if I can find a book from which they can extract the simple and useful notions necessary to understand the memory diseases... Unfortunately I had nothing to offer, all the edited books (at least in our country) presented this vast and still controversial pathology at a scientific level. Therefore, I felt obligated to note on paper, as intelligibly as possible (while still trying not to lose the exact, professional side) the essential elements related to "Alzheimer's". This is how this writing came to be, which flowed normally as the most frequent questions asked of me throughout time. As any new book, it requires changes and improvements after the suggestions and criticism of its readers, this being the reason why the first edition of the book was printed in a limited number of copies.

I do not want to end this EPILOGUE without reminding, once again, that any disturbance of memory, thinking, reasoning and behaviour which have the onset at a mature age must send the respective person to a routine checkup at a specialist in memory diseases!

Finally, I want to thank everyone who has been involved in this effort, my family, who has been the first reader and editor of this book, those who have worked to edit it, and last but not least, those who have influenced my medical career until now.

Appendices

Appendix 1 – Cerebral structures involved in the coginitive process

Structure	Function
Frontal Cortex	Long term memory, activation
Hippocampus	Spatial memory
Amygdala	"Affective" memory
Enthorinal cortex	Visual memory
Diencephalon	Logical memory
The reticular activating system	Wakefulness, alertness, concentration

Appendix 2 - Neurocognitive Domains (adapted from DSM V

Cognitive domains	*Examples of symptoms*	*Specific assessments*
Complex attention (sustained, distributive, selective attention and information processing speed).	Minor cognitive disorder: difficulty (delay) in carrying out tasks; errors in daily tasks; difficulties in performing several tasks simultaneously (e.g. driving and carrying out a conversation). Major cognitive disorder: major difficulty in responding to multiple stimuli (e.g. conversation, driving, radio); difficulties in short-term memory (phone numbers); trouble in making mental calculations.	- Accomplish two tasks simultaneously. - Time of combining letters and numbers. - Speed of making calculations. - Speed of reaction (pressing a button quickly after hearing a sound). - Maintaining attention in the presence of several stimuli.
Executive functions (planning,	Minor cognitive disorder: difficulty in	- Ability to exit a labyrinth. - Decision-making

working memory, decision making, error correction, mental flexibility)	complex projects; difficulty in resuming an activity interrupted by an unexpected event (a ringing phone); accusing fatigue. **Major cognitive disorder:** dropping complex projects which require extra concentration to complete any task; needs help in making decisions.	in alternative conditions (gambling). - Ability to retain and use a short-term information (reproduction of the letters of a word in the reversed order). - Ability to correct decision errors.
Praxis and motor skills (including visual perception)	**Minor cognitive disorder:** requires additional orientation aids (e.g. maps, notes); lost if not focused; difficulty in parking the car. **Major cognitive disorder:** significant difficulties in performing previously	**Recognition of familiar faces** (friends, actors) or objects. - Ability to differentiate two-

		familiar activities (driving, using various tools); diminished motor skills decrease the levels of light; orientation in a previously familiar environment.	and three-dimensional figures. - Assemble elements (puzzle), drawing, copying by model. - Introduction of objects in a limited space without its visual perception. - Imitating gestures, pantomime (defining an item by ideas expressed through gestures).
	Social cognition	Minor cognitive disorder: Minor cognitive disorder: mild disorders in behavior and attitude; possible change of personality; but decreased empathy and inhibition; subtle episodes of apathy and anxiety. Major cognitive disorder: behavioral	Recognition of emotions (identifying positive or negative emotions in facial expressions). -Assessment of sensitivity to describe situations of social value.

	disorders obvious; lack of modesty and social compassion; persevering in expressing opinions without interest to interlocutors; inadequate decisions (e.g. choice of dressing).	
Learning and memory	Minor cognitive disorder: difficulty in remembering recent events solved by using lists; re-reading and reviewing for remembering the characters of a novel or film; payment of bills already settled. Major cognitive disorder: repetition of conversations at a short time interval; does not hold short list of shopping items.	- Immediate memory: the ability to recognize a word list (similar to working memory (executive functions) - Recent memory: process evaluation of encoding new information (memorizing a short story or diagrams) by: - evoking elements of story words, - or recognition of some of them. - Semantic memory: helpful in memorizing facts. -

		Autobiographical memory.
Language	Minor cognitive disorder: difficulty in finding words (memory lapse); the use of synonyms when needed, avoiding the use of proper names; grammar mistakes in the expression of ideas (misuse of articles, prepositions, tenses and articles). Major cognitive disorder: significant difficulties in using spoken and written language; use pronouns instead of names; forgetting the names of family members or close friends; stereotypes in speech preceding mutism.	- Expressive language: identification of objects in images; verbal fluency. - Grammar and syntax: specific errors during the interview at people with high educational level. - Receptive language: understanding the message; making verbal commands

Appendix 3 – Time evolution of the three main dementia types

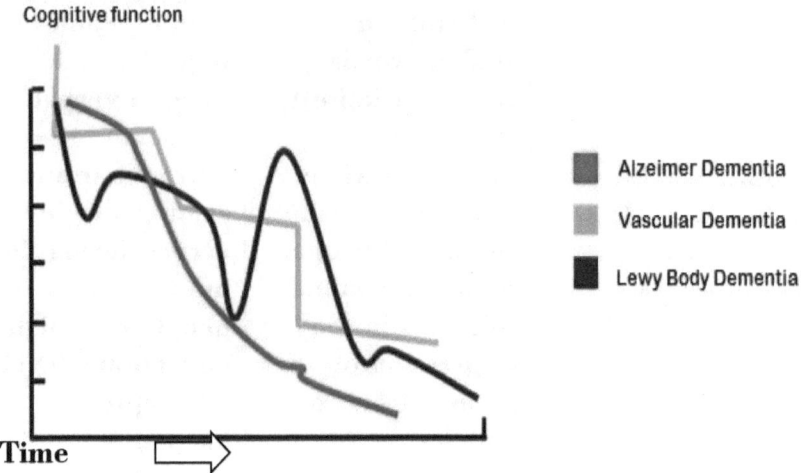

Appendix 4 – The structure of apolipoprotein E correlated with the risk of dementia

APOE correlated with AD

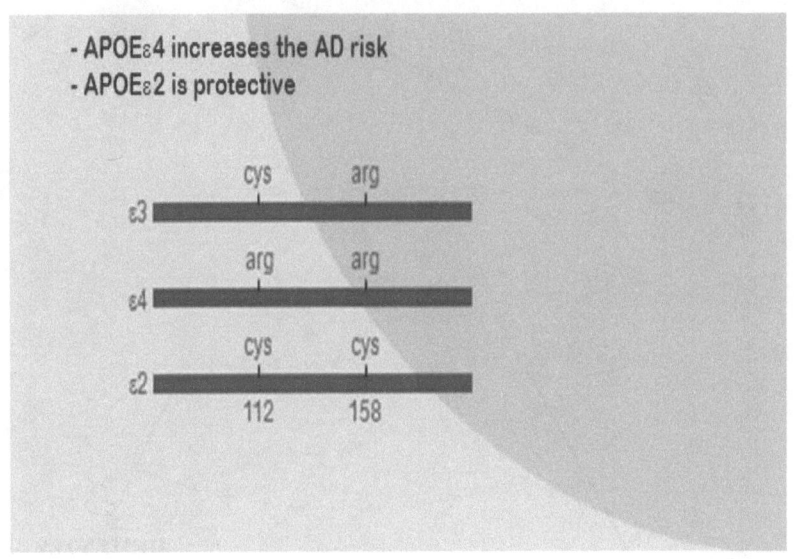

- APOEε4 increases the AD risk
- APOEε2 is protective

Appendix 5 – Scheme of possible pathophysiological evolution in cognitive disorder

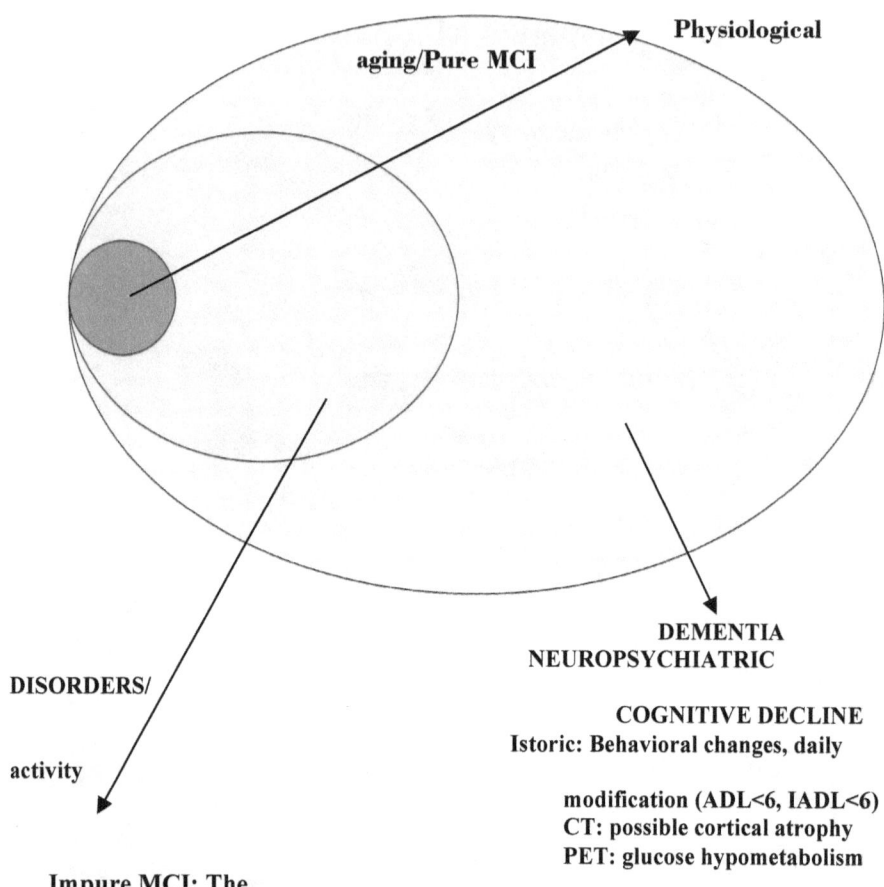

Appendix 6 – Reisberg Scale* (1985)

1. No cognitive decline
2. Very mild cognitive decline (Age Associated
3. Memory Impairment)
4. Mild cognitive decline (Mild Cognitive Impairment)
5. Moderate cognitive decline (Mild Dementia)
6. Moderately severe cognitive decline (Moderate Dementia)
7. Severe cognitive decline (Moderately Severe Dementia)
8. Very severe cognitive decline (Severe Dementia)

Ref: http://www.fhca.org/members/qi/clinadmin/global.pdf

Appendix 7 – ADL/IADL activities of daily living

# ACTIVITIES	ADL	IADL
1.	CORPORAL HYGIENE	TELEPHONE USAGE
2.	DRESSING	SHOPPING
3.	TOILET USAGE	PREPARING MEALS
4.	WALKING	HOUSEWORK
5.	CONTINENCE	LAUNDRY
6.	EATING	HANDLING TRANSPORTATION
7.		HANDLING MEDICATION
8.		MANAGE FINANCES

Appendix 8 – The Metabolic equivalent (MET) for various physical activities

Physical activity	Metabolic equivalent (MET)
Light intensity	**< 3 MET**
Sleeping	0,9
Watching television	1
Writing, typing	1,8
Very slow walking (2,7 km/hour)	2,3
Slow walking (4 km/ora)	2,9
Moderate intensity	**3-6**
Stationary bicycle, very light effort(50 Watt)	3
Walking (4,8 km/ hour)	3,3
Walking (5,5 km/ hour)	3,6
Ciclying (16 km/ hour)	4
Stationary bicycle (100 watts)	5
Vigorous intensity	**>6**
Jogging	7
Rope jumping, basket	8-9

Appendix 9 - Physical effort by the elderly

Effort type	The MET effort maximum intensity for the 65-80 years age group
Very light	< 1.6
Light	1.6 – 3.1
Moderate	3.2 – 4.7
Intense	4.8 – 6.7
Very intense	> 6.8
Maximal	8.0

Appendix 10

Alzheimer Dementia Evolution Phases

PATIENT SYMPTOMS

Normal Phase
- Normal orientation in space, the patient knows own location, date, season or year. Knows geographical location, street, village, etc
- Without memory disorders. They remember easily both recent, as well as past events
- They concentrate without difficulty, converses normally and to the point
- Active person, does not need any help, they can handle themselves in all activities

Mild Phase
- The patient remembers own name, but may have difficulty indicating own occupation, age, etc
- Recent memory is deficient, this being observed in complex discussions
- Occasionally, the patient has difficulty reading, or watching a television program.
- The patient can laugh or cry in an uninhibited or exaggerated manner, to a strong emotional stimulation
- Occasionally disorders of speech occur, such as a limited vocabulary, speech slow, reduced ability to understand other people speech

Medium Phase
- The patient knows what season it is, but not the day of the week, date, month or year
- The patient is confused, in having difficulty to find the way home.
- The patient does not remember the names of family members nor their number
- The patient talks incessantly and gives endless details, but has difficulty in keeping the thoughts and digresses frequently
- The patient reacts in an uninhibited manner at moderate emotional stimulations
- Although active, patient requires constant supervision and help with walking, dressing or personal hygiene

Severe Phase
- The patient is completely disoriented both about themselves as well as spatially and temporally
- Recent memory is completely lost, the patient does not remember specific things at a specific moment
- Reversing the day-night rhythm, nocturnal insomnia and daytime sleepiness
- The power of concentration is so low that it is impossible to hold a full conversation
- Completely dependent from a carer for food and personal hygiene
- The patient shows signs of mental distress, marked by prolonged panic attacks
- All relationships produce a state of increased irritability, which it can even be controlled

Evolution estimate - six years from illness detection in incipient stage — late diagnostic

| Three years | Two years | One year |

©Stănescu et al.

Appendix 11 – Nutritional state clasification as a function of the body mass index

Patient (as function of nutritional state)	Body Mass Index (G/I^2)	Percentual deficit from the ideal weight
Underweight		
Grade 2	<16	- >30
Grade 1	16-17,9	-30 to – 21
SLIM	18 – 19,9	- 20 to – 11
NORMAL	20 - 25	- 10 to + 10
OVERWEIGHT	25,1 – 26,9	+ 11 to + 20
OBESE		
Grade 1	27 – 29,9	+ 21 to + 32
Grade 2	30 – 40	+ 33 to + 77
Grade 3	>40	> 77

Appendix 12 Cognition Tests – Cognitive Tests With Evaluation of Normal/MCI/Dementia Scores

TEST	Assessed Area	SCORE		
		NORMAL	MCI	DEMENTIA
MMSE (Mini MentalState Examination)	Orientation, immediate and short term memory, attention, speaking, executive functions, apraxia	* 27-30 ** 30	* 21-27 **24-30	* <21 ** <24
Clock drawing test	Temporal orientation, executive functions, apraxia	10	7-9	0-6
Verbal fluency	Memory, attention, concentration	>15	>8	<10
Rey–Osterrieth complex figure - Copy	Visuoconstructive praxis, attention, strategy	18/18	16-18	<16
Rey–Osterrieth complex figure - Reproduction	Short term memory, apraxia, strategy	>14	>8	<8
Grober Buscke Test	Short term memory, attention, concentration	>10	>6	<8

References

1. Adams, R. et al. (1997). *Principles of Neurology, 6th edition,* McGraw-Hill Companies, International Edition, ISBN 0-07-114836-1.

2. Nussbaum, A. (2013). *The pocket Guide to the DSM-5™ Diagnostic Exam,* Amazon Edition.

3. Leon, M.J., Convit, A., Wolf, O.T., Tarshish, C.Y., DeSanti, S., Rusinek, H., Tsui, W., Kandil, E., Scherer, A.J., Roche, A., Imossi, A., Thorn, E., Bobinski, M., Caraos, C., Lesbre, P., Schlyer, D., Poirier, J., Reisberg, B., Fowler, J., "Prediction of cognitive decline in normal elderly subjects with 2-[(18)F]fluoro-2-deoxy-D-glucose/poitron-emission tomography (FDG/PET)", in *Proc Natl Acad Sci USA.* 2001 Sep 11; 98(19):10966-71.

4. Jack, C.R. Jr., Petersen. R.C., Grundman, M., Jin, S., Gamst, A., Ward, C.P., Sencakova, D., Doody, R.S., Thal, L.J., Members of the Alzheimer's Disease Cooperative Study (ADCS). "Longitudinal MRI findings from the vitamin E and donepezil treatment study for MCI", in *Neurobiol Aging.* 2008 Sep; 29(9):1285-95.

5. Visser, P.J., Scheltens, P., Verhey, F. R. J., Schmand, B., Launer, L.J., Jolles, J., Jonker, C. (1999). "Medial temporal lobe atrophy and memory dysfunction as predictors for dementia in subjects with mild cognitive impairment", in *J Neurol,* 246, 477-485.

6. Snowdon, D.A., Kemper, S.J., Mortimer, J.A., Greiner, L.H., Wekstein, D.R., Marksebery, W.R. "Linguistic ability in early life and cognitive function and Alzheimer's disease in late life: findings from the Nun Study", in *JAMA* 1996; 275:528–532.

7. D. L. Bachman et al., "Prevalence of dementia and probable senile dementia of the Alzheimer type in the Framingham Study", in *Neurology,* January 1992, vol. 42 no. 1115.

8. Zaldy S. Tan et al., "Thyroid Function and the Risk of Alzheimer's Disease: The Framingham Study", in *Archives of Internal Medicine,* 2008 Jul 28; 168(14): 1514–1520.

9. Carl W. Cotman et al., "Exercise and time-dependent benefits to learning and memory", in *Neuroscience*. 2010 May 19; 167(3): 588–597.

10. Sperling, R.A., Aisen, P.S., Beckett, L.A., Bennett, D.A., Craft, S., "Toward defining the preclinical stages of Alzheimer's disease: Recommendations from the National Institute on Aging-Alzheimer's Association workgroups on diagnostic guidelines for Alzheimer's disease", in *Alzheimers Dement*. 2011 May; 7(3): 280–292.

11. Jian Xu et al., "Inhibitor of the Tyrosine Phosphatase STEP Reverses Cognitive Deficits in a Mouse Model of Alzheimer's Disease", in *PLoS Biol*. 2014 Aug; 12(8): e1001923.

12. Babb, A., "Mediterranean Diet May Help Alzheimer's Patients Live Longer", https://www.aan.com/pressroom/home/pressrelease/541 [retrieved September 14, 2017].

www.ingramcontent.com/pod-product-compliance
Lightning Source LLC
Chambersburg PA
CBHW020900180526
45163CB00007B/2571